T0331685

THE LIFE OF THE HEROIN USER

Typical Beginnings, Trajectories and Outcomes

INTERNATIONAL RESEARCH MONOGRAPHS IN THE ADDICTIONS (IRMA)

Series Editor
Professor Griffith Edwards
National Addiction Centre
Institute of Pyschiatry, London

Volumes in this series present important research from major centres around the world on the basic sciences, both biological and behavioural, that have a bearing on the addictions. They also address the clinical and public health applications of such research. The series will cover alcohol, illicit drugs, psychotropics and tobacco. It is an important resource for clinicians, researchers and policy-makers.

Also in this series:

Mortality amongst Illicit Drug Users: Epidemiology, Causes and Intervention
Shane Darke, Louisa Degenhardt, Richard Mattick
ISBN 9780521855068

Treatment Matching in Alcoholism
Edited by Thomas F. Babor, Frances K. Del Boca
ISBN 9780521177269

Cannabis Dependence: Its Nature, Consequences and Treatment
Edited by Roger Roffman, Robert S. Stephens, Foreword by G. Alan Marlatt
ISBN 9780521891363

Gambling as an Addictive Behaviour: Impaired Control, Harm Minimisation, Treatment and Prevention
Mark Dickerson, John O'Connor
ISBN 9780521847018

Circles of Recovery: Self-Help Organizations for Addictions
Keith Humphreys
ISBN 9780521176378

A Community Reinforcement Approach to Addiction Treatment
Edited by Robert J. Meyers, William R. Miller
ISBN 9780521026345

Cannabis and Cognitive Functioning
Nadia Solowij
ISBN 9780521024808

Alcohol and the Community: A Systems Approach to Prevention
Harold D. Holder
ISBN 9780521035040

THE LIFE OF THE HEROIN USER

Typical Beginnings, Trajectories and Outcomes

SHANE DARKE

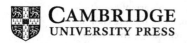
CAMBRIDGE
UNIVERSITY PRESS

CAMBRIDGE
UNIVERSITY PRESS

University Printing House, Cambridge CB2 8BS, United Kingdom

One Liberty Plaza, 20th Floor, New York, NY 10006, USA

477 Williamstown Road, Port Melbourne, VIC 3207, Australia

314-321, 3rd Floor, Plot 3, Splendor Forum, Jasola District Centre, New Delhi - 110025, India

79 Anson Road, #06-04/06, Singapore 079906

Cambridge University Press is part of the University of Cambridge.

It furthers the University's mission by disseminating knowledge in the pursuit of education, learning and research at the highest international levels of excellence.

www.cambridge.org
Information on this title: www.cambridge.org/9781107000636

First published 2011

A catalogue record for this publication is available from the British Library

Library of Congress Cataloging in Publication data
Darke, Shane.
The life of the heroin user: typical beginnings, trajectories and outcomes / Shane Darke.
      p.   cm. – (International research monographs in the addictions)
Includes bibliographical references and index.
ISBN 978-1-107-00063-6 (hardback)
   1. Heroin abuse.   2. Heroin abuse–Treatment.   3. Substance abuse.
   4. Substance abuse–Treatment.   I. Darke, Shane.   II. Title.   III. Series.

HV5822.H4D367 2011
362.29′3–dc22   2011012970

ISBN 978-1-107-00063-6 Hardback

To Skye, Jessica and Lilly.

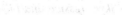

Contents

Contents

Tables

Foreword

This book exemplifies what the IRMA monograph series seeks to achieve in the service of its international readership. It comprehensively and critically reviews an important area of addiction research and offers conclusions of wide relevance to the policy arena. Importantly, it tells us what is unknown or uncertain as well as what is today confidently known, and it offers thinking which will help set further research agendas. This is a book which expertly and in fair-minded fashion is written exactly to meet a contemporary need.

That Shane Darke has found time to author this book despite the demands of a busy and highly productive research career puts us much in his debt. Besides due acknowledgement at the individual level and an expression of admiration toward NDARC (an Australian research centre of high international standing), I see this latest contribution to the IRMA project as speaking to the quality and maturity very generally of the enterprise which is addiction research and its claim to policy relevance.

Griffith Edwards,
Series Editor

Preface

Why write a book on the life of a heroin user? After working in the field of heroin dependence for a quarter of a century, to some extent my fellow researchers and I have grown up with the heroin epidemic. We have seen the impact that the drug makes upon lives. An enormous amount has been written about heroin use, and some excellent longitudinal studies have been conducted. No one, however, has attempted to present a complete lifecycle of heroin use. The picture of this cycle has been building up in my mind across the years. It was time to reflect on what we have learnt, and to produce a single volume that addresses issues that pertain to all aspects and stages of the heroin user's life. In doing so I had a number of questions in mind, with answers that lay in many diverse places in the literature. What is the family background of the typical heroin user? Were their parents drug users? What are their childhood experiences, and how do they relate to later life? How do they get into drugs? Does treatment work? Do people mature out? It seemed to me that synthesising this wide-ranging literature into a single volume might have potentially enormous benefits for researchers, clinicians, relatives of users and those who simply wish to know more about this major public health problem. It is my sincere hope that readers of this book will find the answers to such questions.

It is appropriate for me to acknowledge the enormous assistance that I have received in writing this book. Firstly, the research for the book was funded by the Australian Government Department of Health and Agein. On a personal level, I would like to express my great thanks to Professor Griffith Edwards, the doyen of our field, for his inspiration and support across the years. For their wonderful support of this project, I would also like to thank Kevin Barnes, Matt Berninger, David Bowie, Chiara Bucello, Kate Clowes, Jessica Darke, Lilly Darke, Louisa Degenhardt, Wayne Hall, Martin Iguchi, Mary Kumvaj, Skye McDonald, Joanne Ross, Rachel Taylor and Michelle Torok.

Shane Darke
January 2011

1

Heroin and addict 'careers'

1.1 Introduction

The opiates, the class of drugs of which heroin is a member, carry by far the
highest burden of disease of any drug of dependence and are, worldwide, one
of the leading public health problems. They have an extremely long history in
human civilisation across the globe, extending back at least 6000 years. While
opiate dependence has long been recognised, in the last century this problem
dramatically transformed and expanded following the twin developments of
heroin and the intravenous syringe. We were no longer talking of the more
genteel days of sipping laudanum (tincture of opium, suspended in alcohol).
Injecting opiate use has gone on to consume massive amounts of resources in
health and legal resources across the world. The opioids (a term which
includes both natural opiates and synthetic analogues) are, of course, a core
component of the medical armoury, and have relieved enormous suffering
throughout the course of human civilisation. In the early twenty-first century,
however, heroin and other opiates are also responsible for large-scale mortality and untold misery.

One of the major characteristics of heroin dependence is its remarkably
persistent nature. Terms such as *'chronically relapsing disorder'*, *'lifelong
condition'*, *'chronic illness'* and *'disease'* have been employed in attempts to
capture this perseverance. Of course, this is not to say once a user always a
user. Rather, it is to characterise heroin dependence as a long, difficult battle
for many affected by it. Despite the fact that clinicians and researchers have
long been aware of the extended nature of the problem, it is surprising how
little has been written on the lifecycle, or natural history, of the heroin user.
Of course, there are notable exceptions, such as the pioneering work of David
Nurco and colleagues (Nurco *et al.*, 1981), the oral history of David Courtwright and colleagues (Courtwright *et al.*, 1989) and the more recent work on

trajectories of Yih Ing Hser (Hser *et al.*, 2007a,b). There are a number of possible reasons for this. Firstly, the explosion of heroin use as a major public health concern in western industrialised societies is a phenomenon that arose in the second half of the twentieth century. Those users from the first large-scale heroin epidemics of the 1960s and 1970s are now in their sixth decade and beyond. It is only now that we are seeing the totality of the picture across decades of the lives of individuals and cohorts. Secondly, despite all we know about the intractability of the problem, the public image of the heroin user is of a young person. The idea of people who continue use into their 50s and 60s does not accord well with this image. As we shall see, this image could not be further from the truth. Finally, there is the 'who cares' factor. The concept of young lives at risk carries some cachet. After all, who would not want to save young lives from death and ruin? Old users at risk does not carry quite the same urgency. The irony here is that, clinically, they are at far *greater* risk than their younger counterparts. They are sicker, die at disproportionately higher rates and have generally lived long lives burdened by psychopathology, incarceration and self-harm.

An understanding of the origins and trajectories of heroin use clearly would be valuable in informing interventions. In this book I will attempt to provide a cradle to grave examination of the lives of heroin, and other opioid, users. Where do heroin users come from? How do they get into heroin? Why do they get into heroin? What happens to them? Can their trajectories be changed? In attempting to characterise the life of a dependent opiate user, I will, by necessity, be wielding a rather broad brush. Needless to say, people differ from each other and from society to society, and heroin users are no different in this respect. There are, however, remarkable similarities across cultures in the clinical picture presented by heroin users. It is to these differences and commonalties across the life course that we will address our attention.

In this chapter we will examine the class of opioids themselves, the prevalence of their use, their dependence liability, the harms and costs of opioid use and introduce the concept of an addict 'career'.

1.2   What are the opioids?

Before we begin to examine the lifecycle of the heroin user, we need to first describe what the opioids are, and what their primary positive and negative effects are upon users. The opioids are a class of drugs that include the natural products of the opium poppy *(Papaver somniferum)*, and synthetic compounds derived from it. The term describes any of the narcotic opioid alkaloids found as natural products in the opium poppy plant, as well as many semi-synthetic chemical derivatives (European Monitoring Centre on Drugs and Drug Addiction (EMCDDA), 2010). In addition to heroin, the class includes drugs such as morphine, codeine, methadone, oxycodone and fentynyl. They may also be classified as 'narcotics' or 'narcotic analgesics' (a type of analgesic acting on the central nervous system) due to their soporific and pain relief properties. Although the term 'opiate' is often used as a synonym for opioid, the term is properly limited to only the natural alkaloids found in the resin of the opium poppy. The two major production areas for both opium and heroin are south-west Asia (the 'Golden Crescent', centred on Afghanistan and Pakistan) and south-east Asia (the 'Golden Triangle, centred on Myanmar and Laos) (United Nations Office of Drug Control (UNOCD), 2009). Heroin from south-west Asia is typically brown in colour, and is in the form of a free base. In contrast, south-east Asian heroin is typically a white powder in the form of a hydrochloride salt. Smaller cultivation of opium poppies also occurs in South America, most notably Columbia and Mexico.

Opiates have a long history of both medicinal and recreational use, dating back to at least the Sumerian civilisation of 4000BC (Friedman *et al.*, 1996). The nineteenth century saw a large increase in the use of these drugs due to three key events that were to have lasting and pervasive effects: the isolation of morphine, the invention of the hypodermic syringe and, of particular import, the synthesis of heroin (diacetylmorphine) in 1874. Indeed, heroin was sold as an over-the-counter cough suppressant between 1898 and 1910. The name derives from the German word *'heroisch'* (heroic), which has proved to be sadly ironic as heroin epidemics swept the world over the subsequent century, with attendant pain and misery. There is little that could be counted as heroic about this drug.

What do these drugs do? One of the primary clinical characteristics of opioids is that they produce analgesia, thus the term 'narcotic analgesics'. As noted above, opioids also suppress the cough reflex, and are used in a variety of over-the-counter cough medicines. Opioids act as agonists for a complex group of neuroreceptors (the μ, κ and δ subtypes) that are normally acted upon by endorphins, the body's endogenous opioids. Apart from analgesia, opioids induce drowsiness and sleep. Indeed, the intoxicated heroin user is often referred to as being 'on the nod'. More importantly, from our perspective, opioids produce a sense of euphoria and detachment. These effects are rapid. After ingestion, heroin (diacetylmorphine) is rapidly hydrolysed to 6-monoacetylmorphine, which in turn is hydrolysed to morphine (the main active metabolite) (Goodman & Gilman, 1996). Following heroin injection, diacetylmorphine crosses the blood–brain barrier within 20 seconds. This rapid effect is referred to by users as the 'rush', and is one of the major features of injection as a route of administration. The 'rush' consists of feelings of warmth and pleasure, followed by a long period of sedation. While injection is associated with the most rapid onset of effects, smoking heroin produces an effect that is almost as rapid. Heroin is mainly excreted in the urine as free and conjugated morphine. The plasma half-life of morphine is about 120 minutes. Longer acting opioids such as methadone (12–18 hours) and buprenorphine (24–60 hours) have substantially longer half-lives which is why, as we will see in later chapters, they are used as substitute maintenance drugs for the treatment of heroin dependence. The longer half-life also means that their effects, positive and negative, are more prolonged than that of heroin.

Whilst opioids are associated with considerable pleasure in their subjective effects, they have a number of serious negative sequelae. Use of the drugs, at least prior to the development of tolerance, produces nausea and vomiting. The novice user has to work through these effects to become the long-term user we discuss in this book. There is also decreased motility in the gastro-intestinal tract, resulting in chronic constipation. Indeed, the great poet Coleridge, dependent upon laudanum, was facetiously described as a stranger to the toilet. The major clinically significant negative effect of the opioids is that they are central nervous system (CNS) respiratory depressants (Karch, 2009). Respiration rates are suppressed, even amongst the tolerant and, in overdose may decline to just four breaths per minute, if the person still lives. The cardinal signs of opioid toxicity are the so-called 'diagnostic triad': reduced level of consciousness (from drowsiness to coma), pinpoint pupils and a depressed rate of respiration. Cyanosis, hypotension, bradycardia, hypothermia may also be present. Death is usually due to respiratory failure, although cardiac arrest may occur due to myocardial oxygen deprivation (Goodman & Gilman, 1996).

One of the major sequelae of opioid use of any kind is the development of a dependence syndrome, including physical and psychological aspects (American Psychiatric Association (APA), 2000; White & Irvine, 1999). Signs and symptoms include: increased tolerance, continued use despite physical and/or psychological problems engendered by use and a persistent desire to cut down or control opioid use. The abrupt cessation of use in tolerant subjects leads to characteristic withdrawal symptoms that include rhinorrhoea ('runny nose'), diarrhoea, nausea, muscle spasm and anxiety.

To some extent the route of heroin administration is determined by the geographical source of the drug. The brown powder from south-west Asia may readily be 'smoked' by heating the powder on a metal foil above a flame and inhaling the vapour (Strang *et al.*, 1997). This is known as 'chasing the dragon', a reference to 'chasing' the trail of vapour fumes that emanate from the heated heroin. Brown heroin may be injected, but as it is insoluble in water it first must be dissolved in citric or ascorbic acid, such as lemon juice. The white powder from south-east Asia is soluble in water, and may be dissolved directly in water for injection. It may be smoked, but is not as amenable for this purpose as the brown heroin from the Golden Crescent.

Methadone is dispensed in oral syrup and tablet forms. For maintenance treatment, the syrup preparation is predominant. While usually taken orally, the injection of the syrup by illicit drug users has been documented (Darke *et al.*, 1996a; Humeniuk *et al.*, 2003). Buprenorphine is dispensed as a sublingual tablet for oral ingestion. As with methadone, however, the injection of these tablets has been noted (Mattick *et al.*, 2009). Finally, the other opioid of particular note for this book, oxycodone, is also a tablet-form preparation and, again injection has been noted (Darke *et al.*, 2011).

1.3 How common is heroin use?

Compared with other illicit drugs, such as cannabis, the prevalence of opioid use is relatively low. It is currently estimated that, globally, between 15 and 21 million people aged between 15 and 64 years used opioids in the preceding year (UNOCD, 2009). This translates to between 0.3% and 0.5% of the global population. Rates appear to be highest per capita in Europe (0.6%–0.7%), followed by the Americas and Oceania (0.4%), Africa (0.2%–0.5%) and Asia (0.3%–0.5%). As the proportions of users indicate, opioid use is a truly international phenomenon. Around half (approximately 12 million) of the world's opioid users live in Asian countries (UNOCD, 2009). The next largest population is found in Europe (approximately 4 million), followed by Africa (3 million), the Americas (2.3 million) and Oceania (90 000). It should be noted that there is a consistent gender bias in the prevalence of opioid use, with males approximately twice as likely to be using these drugs (UNOCD, 2009).

Heroin constitutes a large proportion of global opioid use, with approximately 9 million estimated users, or approximately 0.2% of the global population aged 15 to 64 years (UNOCD, 2009). Recent use estimates in some major heroin markets include the United Kingdom (0.1%), the United States (0.2%) and Australia (0.2%). As with the other opioids, the use of heroin is male dominated, as seen in national surveys, street users and treatment samples. Indeed, it is one of the most robust findings of the literature that males constitute approximately two-thirds of lifetime, and current, heroin users.

It should be borne in mind that the illicit opioid market is dynamic, and that use patterns may vary significantly across time. In recent years there has been considerable concern, particularly in the United States, about the abuse of oxycodone, with substantial increases in sales, and deaths attributed to the drug (Carise *et al.*, 2007; Cicero *et al.*, 2005; Forrester, 2007). Indeed, oxycodone deaths in the USA have grown to exceed those due to heroin or cocaine. The dramatic increase in oxycodone use appears to have been driven by a mixture of older, chronic pain patients and younger, illicit opioid users (Carise *et al.*, 2007; Darke *et al.*, 2011).

1.4   The dependence liability of heroin

Heroin and other opioids may result in a dependence syndrome, characterised by a cluster of cognitive, behavioural and physiological symptoms that include tolerance, withdrawal and a persistent desire to cut down (APA, 2000). The most important clinical point to note is that the person continues to use, despite significant drug-related problems (APA, 2000). How likely is it, that once having used opioids, the individual will become dependent upon them? This probability is known as the dependence (or abuse) liability of a substance. Furthermore, how does this liability compare to those of other substances? Despite the salience of heroin and the other opioids as a major clinical and public health issue, surprisingly little work has been conducted on the transition between use and dependence (Anthony *et al.*, 1994; Gable, 1993; Gossop *et al.*, 1992; Robins, 1993; Van Etten & Anthony, 1999). We must commence with opportunities for drug use and the uptake of the drug on offer. Van Etten & Anthony (1999) reported that 20% of those who had an opportunity to use heroin did so, and 17% did so within 12 months of the initial offer. Males were twice as likely as females to have had an opportunity to use heroin. Interestingly, there were no sex differences in the likelihood of use once an opportunity arose, with 18% of males and 26% of females using after being given an opportunity. The authors argued that gender differences in the epidemiology of heroin use are due to opportunity, and *not* due to any differences in susceptibility in the transition to use.

Use is one thing, but the transition to regular use and dependence is quite another. The most influential paper on this issue is that of Anthony *et al.*

(1994), based upon retrospective data collected from the US National Comorbidity Survey. The authors estimated that approximately one in four who used heroin would develop dependence upon the drug. Again, as was seen for opportunity and use, it was notable that there were no differences between males and females in the proportions who developed dependence. Again, once use occurs, females are as likely as males to become heroin dependent. Differences in the gender proportions of users simply reflect opportunity and uptake *per se*, not any differential dependence liability. Of all the drug classes analysed by the authors, heroin was second in dependence liability, with only tobacco having a higher liability of approximately one in three. In contrast, cocaine (17%), alcohol (15%), methamphetamine (11%) and cannabis (9%) were all substantially *lower* in their abuse liability than heroin. Not only is use associated with a substantial risk of future dependence, the risk is higher than for almost all other substances. It should be noted that the incredibly high mortality rates associated with opioids, which we discuss throughout this book, means that the estimates of dependence liability are probably conservative. A great many users who have tried heroin, become dependent and died will not by definition be interviewed in studies of this type. The more marginalised the user population, the more conservative these estimates are likely to be, as dependent heroin users are difficult to contact and interview for large-scale household surveys.

The Vietnam war of the 1960s and 1970s provided an unusual opportunity to examine heroin dependence liability, as cheap heroin was widely available to troops stationed in Vietnam (Robins, 1993). Robins (1993) reported that 40% of US veterans had used opiates whilst in Vietnam, with 20% reporting having become 'addicted' to the drug. The rate here is thus one in two. Clearly, however, this is not a population of street users. These veterans were exposed to high levels of trauma and sheer boredom. Higher rates of use, and the transition to dependence, would both be expected in a combat setting.

An alternative way of examining dependence liability is by measuring the dependence potential and harms associated with a drug (Gable, 1993; Morgan *et al.*, 2010; Nutt *et al.*, 2007, 2010; van Amsterdam *et al.*, 2010). Gable (1993) reported that injected heroin had the greatest risk of dependence and lethality. Opium and morphine were rated next highest in terms of lethality and dependence risk. The lowest risks were associated with cannabis and psilocybin (an hallucinogenic). Similar work conducted by Nutt *et al.* (2007), Morgan *et al.* (2010) and van Amsterdam *et al.* (2010) produced results consistent with these data. The authors examined the physical harms, dependence potential and social harms associated with a number of drug classes.

In terms of all three dimensions of harm, heroin was rated the highest risk. Its dependence risk was rated significantly higher than other widely used illicit drugs such as cocaine and methamphetamine. Similarly, Gossop *et al.* (1994) compared the dependence levels of polydrug users, using an identical dependence scale for each drug class. Heroin dependence varied by route of administration, with injecting associated with the highest levels of dependence. Importantly, and consistent with both Gable (1983) and Nutt *et al.* (2007), heroin dependence levels were significantly higher than those of cocaine and methamphetamine.

Overall, heroin and the other opioids appear to have extremely high dependence liabilities. A likely conservative estimate that one in four who use heroin will develop dependence is certainly pause for thought. Moreover, the dependence liability of the opioids appear higher than those seen for the other major illicit drugs. *Any* use of heroin presents a high risk for dependence. It is this dependence liability that makes the drug such an intractable clinical problem, as we will see in subsequent chapters.

1.5   The major harms of heroin use

The use of heroin and the other opioids is not common, certainly when compared to the use of other illicit drugs such as the psychostimulants and cannabis. Why then, if the number of users is relatively low, are they of such clinical and public health importance? We will discuss the harms of heroin use in detail in subsequent chapters, so at this stage we will only briefly outline them to illustrate the potential for harm to the individual, and how this costs the societies in which they live.

Of illicit drugs, the opioids carry the highest degree of harm and, proportionally, the highest demand for treatment (Darke *et al.*, 2007a; UNOCD, 2009). These harms are expressed in the extremely high rates of premature death seen amongst heroin and other opioid users. Indeed, mortality rates typical of the elderly are one of the defining characteristics of dependent users (Darke *et al.*, 2007a). The major harms associated with regular use include the direct effects of the drugs themselves, serious and often life-threatening psychopathology, and the indirect effects such as criminality and social marginalisation that arise from use. Many of these effects are due to the high dependence liability of heroin discussed above, and the consequent longevity of dependence in individuals. Indeed, dependence can be viewed as one of the most serious harms of opioid use, and of heroin use in particular. It is from this characteristic that all else typically flows.

The other major direct harm of opioid use is the risk of overdose. Overdose is a major contributor to premature death, and non-fatal overdose is associated with a range of serious health sequelae, including brain damage and cognitive impairment (Darke *et al.*, 2007a). As we will see, heroin users also have very poor general health. Much of this relates to injection as a route of administration, and to viral transmission through the sharing of injecting equipment. There are also direct negative health effects from injecting or smoking these drugs, including vascular collapse and pulmonary disease.

The mental health of heroin users is also extremely poor. Indeed, it appears to be even poorer than their generally poor physical health. At least half of any group of heroin users will qualify for a psychiatric diagnosis other than drug dependence, with the most commonly diagnosed disorders being mood, anxiety and personality disorders (Brienza *et al.*, 2000; Kidorf *et al.*, 2004; Teesson *et al.*, 2005). As with their physical health, the burden of psychological disease amongst heroin users is many times that of the general population. Indeed, the treatment of comorbid psychopathology is one of the major challenges that faces drug treatment agencies.

The use of illicit opioids, such as heroin, is an expensive business. The regular heroin user is highly likely to be involved in frequent criminal activity. As we shall see in Chapter 5, approximately half to three-quarters of regular heroin users have a current involvement in crime, apart from the use of illegal drugs (Darke *et al.*, 2010e; Haasen *et al.*, 2007; Van der Zanden, 2007). Not surprisingly, almost all users who have been using for any length of time will have a conviction record, and at least half have been incarcerated (Bargagli *et al.*, 2006; Darke & Ross, 2001; Lofwall *et al.*, 2005). Apart from crime, a great many female users perform high levels of sex work, as do some male users, exposing them to high risks of violence and blood-borne viral infection (Maher *et al.*, 2002; Spital *et al.*, 2003). Involvement in illicit drug use, crime and sex work exposes heroin users to high levels of traumatic injury and, indeed, trauma is a major cause of death amongst users (Darke *et al.*, 2007a).

Finally, the social profile of users is extremely poor. Educational attainment is low, unemployment close to universal and financial problems are the norm (Azim *et al.*, 2008; Galea *et al.*, 2003; Neale & Robertson, 2005; Ross *et al.*, 2005). This is a highly disadvantaged, and socially marginalised, group with a large burden of disease.

The general picture seen here, and elaborated upon in ensuing chapters, is of a highly dysfunctional and ill group of people. The picture is a long way from the so-called *'heroin chic'* image beloved by advertisers worldwide in the mid-1990s. This was a false image built upon a heady mixture of ignorance and stupidity. There is nothing chic about a life of dependence, illness, incarceration and premature death. The life comes with serious cost to individuals and their families. It also comes at great cost to society, as we shall now see.

1.6   Costs to society

As we have seen, the harms associated with heroin dependence are substantial, and completely out of proportion to the prevalence of their use. It should thus not surprise that these harms come with enormous costs to society, as well as to the individual user. Attempting to define the costs of drug dependence, or of opioid dependence in particular, is fraught with difficulty. There are direct and indirect costs to be considered. The most common framework to evaluate the burden of disease associated with substance use is a 'cost of illness' analysis (Collins *et al.*, 2007; Harwood *et al.*, 1998; Mark *et al.*, 2001; Rehm *et al.*, 2006; Strassels, 2009). Analyses cover three types of costs: (i) direct costs, (ii) indirect costs from loss of output and (iii) psychosocial costs. Factors to be considered include medical care, crime, lost productivity and social welfare (Mark *et al.*, 2001).

The most obvious direct costs of opioid dependence are the costs of treatment and medical care. As noted above, opioids have, proportionally, the highest demand for treatment (UNOCD, 2009). As we will see in subsequent chapters, treatment tends to be protracted and repeated across many enrolments. For outpatient pharmacological interventions, such as methadone, there are the costs of the drugs themselves, as well as the costs of medical practitioners and nursing staff to administer these drugs. Inpatient drug-free residential rehabilitation does not entail medication costs, but does entail the costs of providing beds, food and staff. There are also the medical sequelae of heroin addiction to consider in direct costings. As we have noted, the dependent heroin user is generally in poor health, ambulance callouts for overdoses are common, and rates of blood-borne viral infections requiring hospitalisation and expensive medications are high. Similarly, levels of psychopathology are extraordinarily high, and concomitant treatment of these problems consumes medical resources.

The direct costs of heroin addiction are not restricted to health costs. We must also take into account the direct costs of the criminal behaviours that are commonly conducted to support drug use. As noted above, acquisitive criminal behaviours are common, as are arrests and incarceration. Involved here are the direct costs of crime to the victims, and to the wider society in the form of higher insurance policy costs. There are also the direct costs of law enforcement and of incarceration, the latter of which is particularly expensive.

We must also take into account the indirect costs resulting from loss of output. Essentially, we are talking here about loss of earnings and lost production (Mark *et al.*, 2001). Almost all dependent drug users are unemployed, which means that they are not considered to be economically contributing to production, and have reduced earnings with which to consume goods. There is also the loss of income and productivity in periods of incarceration. The major indirect cost, however, stems from the high rates of mortality amongst opioid users, higher than for any other drug (Darke *et al.*, 2007a). Given the mean age at death is in the early 30s, we are seeing a shortening of life in the order of 40 years (Darke *et al.*, 2007a). This can be viewed as 40 years of lost income and productivity. One measure of loss due to mortality and morbidity is the Disability Adjusted Life Year (DALY), used by the World Health Organization to estimate the global burden of disease (Degenhardt *et al.*, 2004). DALYs are defined as the sum of years of potential life lost due to premature mortality, and the years of productive life lost due to disability. They are thus a combined measure of lost life and disability. In the year 2000 alone, it was estimated that over 6.87 million DALYs were attributable to illicit drug use, which represents 0.8% of *all* global DALYs for that year (Degenhardt *et al.*, 2004). Whilst drug specific estimates have not been made to date, death rates due to overdose and disease amongst heroin and other opioid users suggest that these drugs contribute a substantial proportion of these DALYs.

Finally, there are social welfare costs that stem from all of the above. Long-term users are usually unemployed, in marginal health and are on some form of government benefit. There are also the more intangible costs of a low quality of life for the dependent user and their families (Collins *et al.*, 2007). Opioid dependence is a major social problem. It is not surprising that it comes with substantial social costs.

Given all of the above, we would expect the costs to society to be substantial. We would not be disappointed in this assumption. Mark *et al.*, (2001) estimated that in the USA, for the year 1996 alone, the annual cost of heroin dependence was US$22 billion, a not insignificant amount for a single country in a single year. Proportionally, it was estimated that productivity losses accounted for half of this amount, crime for a quarter, medical care for a quarter and social welfare for 0.5%. White *et al.* (2005) estimated that the annual direct health costs of an opioid abuser in the USA were eight times those of non-abusers. In Australia, with a population of around a twentieth that of the USA, annual costs of illicit drug use are estimated at A$7 billion annually (Collins *et al.*, 2007). In Canada, the comparable figure is C$40 billion (Rehm *et al.*, 2006). We should not, however, restrict estimates to illicit drugs. It was recently estimated that the total annual cost of prescription opioid abuse in the USA was US$9 billion (Strassels, 2009).

Opioid use may not be a common social problem, but it is a very, very expensive one. Independent of the individual suffering involved, the costs to society make opioid dependence a social problem worthy of the closest attention.

1.7   The addict 'career'

Finally, we must introduce the concept of an 'addiction career', which is central to this book. Why do we need to use a term like this, that carries an implication of long-term involvement? As intimated above, and as we shall see in later chapters, heroin dependence is incredibly perseverative, and it is for these reasons it has been characterised as a chronically relapsing disorder or disease. The concept of a use career is a means of capturing this longevity, and the transitions the opioid dependent individual will undergo throughout their life course. An addiction 'career' may be defined as a process in which drug use escalates to more severe levels, with repeated cycles of cessation and relapse occurring over an extended period (Hser *et al.*, 2007a; Nurco *et al.*, 1981). An advantage of conceptualising drug dependence in this manner is that we move from the concept of dependence as an acute disorder, requiring short-term interventions. Dependence is likely to be long term and the problems faced by the user will differ at different stages of their life course. The health and social issues being faced by the 60-year-old dependent user, for instance, are likely to differ substantially from those of the heroin user aged in their 20s.

As others have pointed out (Hser *et al.*, 2007b), the term 'career' carries, inadvertently, an unwanted implication of something to be strived for. A successful career is something society values. This could hardly be said of a successful heroin using career, whatever that could be construed to mean. A lifelong devotion to heroin intoxication will hardly be seen as cause for celebration. An alternative term suggested by some authors in this field is '*drug use trajectory*', a phrase that does not carry such connotations (e.g. Hser *et al.*, 2007b). The concept, however, is identical. We are speaking of the path the person takes in life, in particular, their transitions between life stages and significant turning points, such as treatment entry. The term 'career' derives from criminology, and the concept of the criminal career. The term is probably more apposite to acquisitive crime as a source of income. As Hser *et al.* (2007b) point out, there is also an analogy with disease progression or *'illness careers'*. Indeed, the trajectory of illness (or chronically relapsing condition) is particularly apposite, with analogies to other chronic conditions such as asthma or diabetes. Analyses of illness careers examine symptom onset, disease onset, chronicity, remission, recurrence and recovery. In terms of heroin dependence, the analogous foci are the onset of use, the onset of dependence, duration of use, cessation of use, relapse to use and sustained recovery. In both chronic disease and illicit drug use, contact with treatment services is a crucial component of the life course, and of potential recovery. Of course, many users will also have concomitant criminal and illness careers.

In this book we will examine the life of a 'typical' heroin user from the cradle to the grave. We will examine the gateways into drug and heroin use, typical trajectories of opioid use, transition points such as treatment, relapse, routes out of heroin use and death. Of course, there is no one career or trajectory that will cover the life course of all heroin users. Indeed, a number of different trajectories have been identified (Hser *et al.*, 2007a; Nurco *et al.*, 1981). As noted above, however, there are remarkable similarities in the long-term clinical pictures of opioid users, and of heroin users in particular. For our purposes, it is the long-term heavy user who is of the greatest public health and clinical interest, and who will be the primary focus of this book, although not to the exclusion of other paths. We will examine each life stage of the opioid user, and the issues faced by them at these junctures.

Before moving on, we must briefly address the concept of the high functioning, employed heroin user. I have often heard it argued that there is a hidden group of employed, 'recreational' heroin users that may, indeed, be larger in size than the poorly functioning lower socioeconomic group that is usually seen as 'typical'. I remain extremely sceptical about the existence of this group. They do not turn up at police stations, prison, treatment or as overdose fatalities. The latter is particularly instructive, since for drugs such as cocaine, in which a high functioning group do exist in large numbers in parallel to the lower socioeconomic IDU, the profile of fatal overdoses reflects this (Darke *et al.*, 2005a). Such a group of heroin users will be small in number and, given the above, of no great clinical interest.

Finally, we need to acknowledge some caveats in the data we will be discussing. Firstly, the overwhelming bulk of studies in the literature are from developed countries, particularly those in North America, Europe and Australasia. The picture of opiate abuse in developing countries is far less well documented. Secondly, for logistical reasons, most cohorts have been initially recruited from treatment entrants. They may thus possibly present a poorer long-term profile than the broader heroin using population. We should note, however, that there are great similarities between treatment and non-treatment heroin using populations that give some confidence in the utility of such studies. Finally, there will always be problems that arise from the very facts that heroin use is statistically rare, and that heroin users are a 'hidden' population who use illicit drugs and who may attempt to avoid the public gaze, as seen in the oral histories of long-term users presented by Courtwright *et al.* (1989).

1.8 Summary

The most important points to emerge from this chapter are the high dependence liability of heroin and the other opioids, and the concept of a heroin use career or trajectory. As the term career suggests, and as we will see in later chapters, it is not only the dependence liability of heroin that is of relevance, but the longevity of the addiction careers of many users. It is not for nothing that terms such as *'chronically relapsing disorder'* are employed. One of the reasons why heroin carries the highest burden of disease of any drug is the sheer chronicity of most use careers.

In examining the life course of the heroin user, and what factors may influence their progression to heroin use, we must first study their backgrounds. In the next chapter we will commence our journey through the life of a typical user by focusing on their parents and childhood experiences, and how these factors may influence their development.

> **Key points: Summary of heroin and addict 'careers'**
>
> - Heroin is an opioid, a class of drugs that includes the natural products of the opium poppy and synthetic compounds derived from it. Other opioids include methadone, buprenorphine, oxycodone and fentynyl.
> - Opioids induce analgesia, drowsiness, a sense of euphoria and of detachment. Negative effects include dependence, respiratory depression, nausea and vomiting.
> - Between 15 and 21 million people aged between 15 and 64 years use heroin annually, between 0.3% and 0.5% of the global population.
> - The dependence liability of heroin is second only to tobacco. Approximately one in four people who use the drug will develop dependence.
> - The major harms of heroin dependence include the direct effects of the drugs themselves (e.g. overdose), and indirect effects such as crime and social marginalisation.
> - The costs of heroin dependence include direct costs (e.g. treatment and medical costs), indirect costs from loss of output (e.g. due to mortality, unemployment, incarceration) and psychosocial costs (e.g. social welfare costs, lower quality of life).
> - An addiction 'career' is a process in which drug use escalates to more severe levels, with repeated cycles of cessation and relapse occurring over an extended period. An alternative, and more neutral, term is 'drug use trajectory'.

2

Parents and childhood

2.1 Introduction

Clearly, there was a time in a heroin user's life prior to their use of, and dependence upon, heroin. We will commence our review of the life and trajectories of heroin users by examining their early life experiences. If we are to understand why people become heroin users, how this happens and why their trajectories look like they do, we need to examine their developmental patterns. In this chapter, we will examine the childhood social backgrounds of heroin users, the drug use and psychopathology of their parents, traumatic childhood events, childhood psychopathology and the possible role of genetic predispositions for the development of heroin dependence.

2.2 Social disadvantage

It is well demonstrated that social disadvantage is associated with poorer physical and mental health, including higher rates of depression, cardiovascular disease, lung cancer and mortality (Graham & Power, 2004; Wilkinson & Marmot, 2003). Of particular relevance to this discussion, social disadvantage is associated with higher rates of psychoactive substance use and dependence (Anthony *et al.*, 1994; Daniel *et al.*, 2009; Galea *et al.*, 2003; Hser, 2007; Kandel, 1991; Miech *et al.*, 2005; Spooner & Hetherington, 2004). In examining the role of disadvantage, we may conceptualise it at the level of the community, the family or the individual.

Importantly, the level of disadvantage of a community has a strong association with poorer health and higher rates of substance use disorders (Bobashev & Anthony, 1998; Galea *et al.*, 2004; Petronis *et al.*, 2003; Spooner & Hetherington, 2005; Weatherburn & Lind, 2001). Impoverished social environments tend to have high rates of crime, delinquency and substance availability. There are limited educational opportunities, higher rates of early school leaving, lower levels of employment, higher incarceration rates and higher levels of stress upon individuals and families. We also see lower birth weights, higher rates of child abuse and elevated mortality rates (Bobashev & Anthony, 1998; Galea *et al.*, 2004; Petronis & Anthony, 2003; Spooner & Hetherington, 2004; Weatherburn & Lind, 2001). The general picture is of a clustering in lower socioeconomic communities of social and health problems. This scenario of increased levels of financial and psychological stress, and wider substance availability also represents a clustering of risk factors for drug use. Not surprisingly, given the higher rates of community risk factors, disadvantaged communities have higher rates of initiation into tobacco, alcohol and illicit drug use, and of the development of substance dependence (Bobashev & Anthony, 1998; Daniel *et al.*, 2009; Fergusson & Horwood, 1997; Fite *et al.*, 2009; Galea *et al.*, 2004; Hawkins *et al.*, 1992; Lemstra *et al.*, 2008; Nandi *et al.*, 2010; Petronis & Anthony, 2003; Weatherburn & Lind, 2001). Of particular relevance to this book, the incidence of heroin overdose increases with the poverty of a district (Degenhardt *et al.*, 2011; Galea *et al.*, 2003; Marzuk *et al.*, 1997; Najman *et al.*, 2008). This is a marker both for higher rates of heroin use in poorer communities, and for higher rates of harm in such communities.

We must, however, also consider the disadvantage of the family itself in relation to risk factors for substance use. Child development and health are affected by their family's socioeconomic background, effects that will impact upon their adult lives (Lemstra *et al.*, 2008; Najman *et al.*, 2008). Children from lower socioeconomic background families are more likely to experience childhood abuse and neglect, as well as depression and hopelessness (Galea *et al.*, 2004; Graham & Power, 2004; Poulton *et al.*, 2002). They are also more likely to have parents who smoke and use alcohol and/or illicit drugs (Anthony *et al.*, 1994; Daniel *et al.*, 2009; Hawkins *et al.*, 1992; Hemmingsson *et al.*, 1997; Muntaner *et al.*, 1998). This is demonstrated by the higher rates seen amongst lower socioeconomic families of parental alcoholism, alcohol-related assault, foetal alcohol syndrome, alcohol-related deaths, illicit drug use and lung cancer deaths (Muntaner *et al.*, 1998; Hemmingsson *et al.*, 1997; Hemstrom, 2002; Marzuk *et al.*, 1997; Najman *et al.*, 2008). At the family level, lower socioeconomic children thus have exposure to higher levels of familial risk factors, independent of the status of their community. The longer familial poverty persists, the more persistent are the negative effects (Spooner & Hetherington, 2004). In particular, substance dependence amongst parents is associated with an increased risk of substance dependence amongst their children. Higher rates of childhood abuse and neglect are of particular importance, as we will see below, as they are strongly associated with substance dependence, and with heroin dependence in particular. Not surprisingly, given all of the above, lower socioeconomic family status is associated with higher rates of licit and illicit drug use amongst the children of these families (Daniel *et al.*, 2009; Lemstra *et al.*, 2008).

Finally, at the level of the individual, lower socioeconomic individuals are more likely to have problematic use across a range of substances (Anthony *et al.*, 1994; Hawkins *et al.*, 1992; Hemmingsson *et al.*, 1997; Muntaner *et al.*, 1998). Individual factors such as unemployment and lower educational levels are correlated with the use of illicit drugs such as cannabis, amphetamines and heroin (Kandel, 1991; Kandel *et al.*, 1997; Lynskey & Hall, 2000; Warner *et al.*, 1995). The relevance here is that the cycle is likely to repeat. Thus, the young heroin user is more likely to grow up with disadvantage, which is likely to persist through later life. We will see in later chapters that, as adults, the socioeconomic status of heroin users is generally low, with high rates of unemployment and low educational attainment (cf. Chapter 5). They will thus be likely to provide an environment for *their* children of low socioeconomic status, parental drug use and high rates of abuse, similar to that in which they themselves developed.

The above should *not* be interpreted as indicating that substance use is contained to the poor. This would be an absurd suggestion. There are certainly substance dependence problems in more privileged communities and families. Indeed, young people from such backgrounds are more likely to have money to purchase drugs than those from disadvantaged backgrounds. What is being asserted here is that, like health and social problems more generally, each increment in socioeconomic status reduces the odds of the child becoming substance dependent. Essentially, there is an accretion of risk factors for drug dependence the lower the socioeconomic standing of the community, family and individual.

2.3   Parents of heroin users

2.3.1   Parental substance abuse

We must now briefly examine the parents of heroin users, as parental substance use and abuse is of critical importance in the development of our heroin user (Fergusson *et al.*, 1994b,c,d; Fergusson & Lynskey, 1997; Goodwin *et al.*, 2004; Hser *et al.*, 2007a,b; Lynskey *et al.*, 1994; Ohannessian *et al.*, 2004;

Simons & Giorgio, 2008). There are several reasons for this. Firstly, the children of parents with substance abuse disorders are significantly more likely to develop such disorders themselves. Secondly, such children are significantly more likely to experience childhood abuse. Finally, such children are significantly more likely to develop a range of psychopathology, including mood, anxiety and conduct disorders, which are in themselves related to the development of substance use disorders.

Why do these associations exist? In terms of substance use, there is the possibility of behavioural modelling by children of parental substance use, which increases the risk of adolescent substance use behaviour. Similarly, there is evidence that, if parents hold permissive attitudes towards the use of specific substances by their children, their children will be more likely to use such substances (Hawkins *et al.*, 1992). The link between parental substance abuse and child abuse is, in part, due to increased level of disinhibition and violence associated with the substance dependence of the parents (Athanasiadus 1999; Darke, 2010; Goldstein, 1985; Phillips *et al.*, 2007). Illicit substance use is strongly linked to violent assault, both as perpetrator and as victim (Darke, 2010). Drugs such as alcohol and the psychostimulants are associated with pharmacologically induced violence. Substances such as heroin may not directly induce violence, but heroin dependence involves immersion in a violent sub-culture, as we will see in later chapters. It is thus likely that there will be an environment of family discord, poor behavioural management and/or low levels of family bonding (Hawkins *et al.*, 1992). Finally, given childhood abuse is at higher levels than amongst the children of non-users, we would expect to find higher rates of childhood and adult psychopathology than would be expected. We must also keep in mind that substance dependence is strongly associated with psychopathology and, as we will see below, rates of psychopathology and dysfunction are high amongst parents of heroin users.

There are thus good reasons to suspect that many parents of heroin users will have been substance abusers themselves. As expected, rates of substance abuse amongst the parents of heroin users are consistently high (Table 2.1). In most studies, a third or more of opioid users had at least one substance dependent parent. Reflecting the epidemiology of its use, alcohol dependence is particularly notable. Rates of parental illicit drug use are also high, and may be expected to rise as succeeding generations increase their prevalence of illicit drug use. By way of comparison, population estimates of levels of alcohol dependence are under 2% and drug dependence under 1% (Kessler & Wang, 2008; Slade *et al.*, 2009; Wells *et al.*, 2006). By any standards, rates of substance dependence amongst the parents of heroin users are many

Table 2.1. Substance abuse and psychopathology amongst parents of heroin users

Study	Sample	Substance abuse	Psychopathology and separation
Bailey et al. (1994)	USA. Treatment patients	Alcohol 37%, illicits 18%	–
Chatham et al. (1995)	USA. Methadone patients	–	Pathology: Mother 12%, Father 4%
Chiang et al. (2006)	Taiwan. Young incarcerated heroin users	Illicits 40%	86% single parent families
Conroy et al. (2009)	Australia. Methadone patients	46%	Separation before age 7: 32%
Coviello et al. (2004)	USA. Methadone patients	68%	–
Darke & Ross (2001)	Australia. Methadone patients	57%	Pathology: 22%. Parent absent 37%
Deykin & Buka (1994)	USA. Dependent adolescents	Alcohol 70%, drugs 47%	Pathology: 46%
Hser (2007)	USA. Heroin users	30%. Father alcoholic 14%, Mother 2%	Parents divorced before age 15: 35%
Ohannessian et al. (2004)	USA. General population	Parental problem alcohol use related to alcohol dependence, conduct disorder and depression	–
Pugatch et al. (2001)	USA. Heroin users in detoxification	80%	–
Ravndal et al. (2001)	Norway. Therapeutic community clients	Alcohol 40%, drugs 19%	Pathology: 41%
Rossow & Lauritzen (2001)	Norway. Treatment patients	Alcohol: Father 45%, Mother 43%	Pathology: 10%. Parents divorced before age 16: 47%
Simons & Giorgio (2008)	USA. Treatment entrants	Father 51%, Mother 57%	–
Westermeyer et al. (2001)	USA. Treatment patients	Father 45%, Mother 26%	–

times that of the general population. Again, it should be emphasised that these data are not saying that all heroin users will have substance-abusing parents. Similarly, not all substance-abusing parents will have children who end up as heroin users. It is clear, however, that there is a highly elevated risk for the development of heroin dependence when the person comes from a parental background involving substance abuse.

2.3.2 Parental psychopathology

The second aspect of familial history that is of relevance to our heroin user is parental psychopathology. As we have seen, rates of substance abuse amongst the parents of heroin users are high. We also know that substance dependence is associated with significantly elevated rates of psychopathology. As such, we would expect to see high rates of psychopathology amongst the parents of opioid users. The few studies that have reported on this are consistent with this expectation (Table 2.1). In all studies where it was reported, the mental illness histories of the parents of users are high. In a study my colleagues and I conducted on methadone patients, for instance, one in five patients reported that they had at least one parent whom they know was treated for a psychiatric illness (Darke & Ross, 2001). In studies by Deykin & Buka (1994) and Ravndal *et al.* (2001), nearly half of substance users reported that their parents had been treated for mental health problems. Of course, these are in all probability conservative estimates, as the person may not be aware of psychiatric or psychological treatments received by their parents. The rates of psychiatric illness indicated by these treatment figures is many times what we would expect of the general population (Kessler & Wang, 2008; Slade *et al.*, 2009; Wells *et al.*, 2006).

Parental psychopathology is of great importance, as one of the most robust findings in the psychiatric literature is that mental illness has strong familial relations (APA, 2001; Luthar *et al.*, 1993; Nunes *et al.*, 1998; Wilens *et al.*, 2002). As with the transmission of substance abuse, mental illness in parents tends to beget mental illness in the next generation. As we will see in later chapters, rates of psychopathology amongst adult heroin users are extraordinarily high. Parental psychopathology, as well as drug use, is one of the factors that engenders such high rates. There is, however, likely to be significant family disruption and conflict associated with parental psychopathology, including a higher likelihood of childhood abuse and neglect (cf. Section 2.4). This is particularly likely to be so if the parents are illicit drug users *with* psychopathology. Not surprisingly, high rates of conflict are reported amongst the parents of heroin users (Conroy *et al.*, 2009). Parental separation or absence during childhood also appears to be common amongst heroin users, with a third or more reporting such circumstances (Table 2.1). This is, in and of itself, important as parental separation or absence during childhood is associated with increased risk for mood, conduct and substance use disorders, as well as suicide (Fergusson *et al.*, 1994a; Lipman *et al.*, 2002; Spooner & Hetherington, 2004).

As with parental substance use, we must emphasise that not all heroin users will have had parents with serious psychopathology, and not all parents with psychopathology will have children who end up as heroin users. Parental psychopathology, however, is prevalent in the backgrounds of heroin users, and would appear to increase the risk of heroin dependence in their offspring.

2.4   Genetics and heroin dependence

We have seen that substance use tends to cluster within families, with parental substance dependence increasing the risk of substance use disorders in their children (Fergusson & Lynskey, 1997; Goodwin *et al.*, 2004; Hser *et al.*, 2007a; Ohannessian *et al.*, 2004; Simons & Giorgio, 2008; Tyrfingsson *et al.*, 2010). A great deal of research has gone into the major environmental factors associated with these familial patterns, including community and family disadvantage, parental psychopathology and child abuse. In recent years, however, we have seen a considerable increase in research activity into the possibility of an inherited genetic susceptibility for substance dependence (Agrawal & Lynskey, 2008; Kendler & Prescott, 1998; Tyrfingsson *et al.*, 2010). Research from twin, adoption and family studies certainly suggests that there is a genetic component that does increase the likelihood of dependence on alcohol, cannabis, opioids, hypnosedatives and psychostimulants (Agrawal & Lynskey, 2008; Goldman *et al.*, 2005; Kendler *et al.*, 2003; Tyrfingsson *et al.*, 2010). Importantly, elevated familial risk has also been demonstrated between distant relations who share few environmental commonalities (Agrawal & Lynskey, 2008; Goldman *et al.*, 2005; Kendler *et al.*, 2003; Tyrfingsson *et al.*, 2010). It should be noted that such research is *not* suggesting that those with a genetic predisposition will inevitably develop opioid dependence, merely that they have an elevated risk of doing so.

While there does appear to be some predisposition to opioid dependence, determining the genetic underpinnings for such a vulnerability has proved

Table 2.2. Childhood abuse histories of heroin users

Study	Sample	Sexual abuse	Physical abuse	Emotional abuse	Neglect
Bailey et al. (1994)	USA. Treatment patients	5%	18%	–	–
Bartholomew et al. (2005)	USA. Female methadone entrants	39%	67%	74%	–
Braitstein et al. (2003)	Canada. IDU	24%, M 12% F 33%	–	–	–
Branstetter et al. (2008)	USA. Treatment patients	12%, M 4% F 30%	26%, M 18% F 48%	40%, M 31% F 61%	–
Chiang et al. (2006)	Taiwan. Young incarcerated heroin users	4%	31%	–	16%
Conroy et al. (2009)	Australia. Methadone patients	50%, M 36% F 72% Contact M 7% F 10% Penetration 35%, M 21% F 56%	M 58% F 59%	52%, M 46% F 60%	72%, M 68% F 78%
Darke et al. (2010e)	Australia. Opiate and methamphetamine users	–	48% (all abuse)	–	–
Deykin & Buka (1994)	USA. Dependent adolescents	M 10% F 72%	M 41% F 55%	–	–
Farrugia et al. (in press)	Australia. PTSD and substance use patients	Molested 52%, M 46% F 56% Penetration 34%, M 33% F 35%	32%, M 33% F 31%	–	–
Freeman et al. (2001)	USA. Female partners of IDU	39%	–	–	–

Table 2.2. (contd.)

Study	Sample	Sexual abuse	Physical abuse	Emotional abuse	Neglect
Gilbert et al. (1997)	USA. Female methadone patients	27%	39%	–	–
Gil-Rivas et al. (1997)	USA. Outpatients	39%, M 13% F 61%	55%, M 45% F 62%	–	–
Hartel et al. (2006)	USA. Current drug users	22%, M 15% F 36%	39%, M 39% F 42%	–	–
Heffernan et al. (2000)	USA. Psychiatric admissions	–	60% (physical and/or sexual)	–	–
Hien et al. (2000)	USA. Methadone entrants	23%, M 19% F 27%	17%, M 4% F 29%	–	–
Lau et al. (2005)	Hong Kong. Adolescent heroin users	–	Abused to injury 8%	–	–
Medrano et al. (2002)	USA. Current users	39%, M 23% F 53%	72%, M 73% F 71%	–	–
Ompad et al. (2005)	USA. IDU	12%, M 5% F 30%. Earlier onset of injecting	–	–	–
Ouimette et al. (2000)	USA. Treatment seekers	3%, M 2% F 8%	20%, M 20% F 21%	–	–
Oviedo-Joekes et al. (2011)	Canada. Maintenance patients	20%, M 9% F 36%	43% (M = F)	63% (M = F)	–

Plotzker et al. (2007)	USA. Female IDU	56%	68%	–	–
Ravndal et al. (2001)	Norway. RR clients	25% (high trauma), M 21% F 36%	–	–	–
Rosen et al. (2002)	USA. Treatment seekers	9%, M 8% F 51%	26%, M 25% F 63%	–	–
Rossow & Lauritzen (2001)	Norway. Treatment patients	49%	46%	–	–
Sansone et al. (2009)	Buprenorphine treatment entrants	20%	40%	60%	23%
Simons & Giorgio (2008)	USA. Treatment entrants	F > M	M = F	M = F	M = F
Surratt et al. (2004)	USA. Dependent female sex workers	51%	45%	62%	45%
Triffleman et al. (1995)	USA. Male treatment patients	54%	91%	–	73%
Westermeyer et al. (2001)	USA. Treatment patients	30%, M 23% F 40%	–	–	–
Wu et al. (2010)	USA. Residential patients	48%	49%	66%	17%

difficult (Clarke *et al.*, 2009; De los Cobos 2007; Drakenberg *et al.*, 2006; Glatt *et al.*, 2007; Haile *et al.*, 2008; Kosarac *et al.*, 2008; Lachman *et al.*, 2007; Mayer & Hollt, 2006; Saxon *et al.*, 2005). Not unnaturally, most research to date has focussed on genetic variations in the mu opioid neuro-receptors as the most likely candidates (Clarke *et al.*, 2009; De los Cobos 2007; Drakenberg *et al.*, 2006; Haile *et al.*, 2008; Lachman *et al.*, 2007).

The exact nature of these putative genetic vulnerabilities remains unclear. One line of research has focussed on a possible association between nucleotide polymorphism of the A118G μ receptor gene and risk for opioid dependence (Clarke *et al.*, 2009; De los Cobos 2007; Drakenberg *et al.*, 2006; Haile *et al.*, 2008). It has been hypothesised that variations in the expression of this gene may influence the rapidity of opioid metabolism. Slow opioid metabolisers may well be somewhat protected from opioid dependence, while rapid metabolisers may be at increased risk. Some studies have reported such an association (De los Cobos 2007; Drakenberg *et al.*, 2006; Haile *et al.*, 2008). Others have reported such associations, but that they were specific to gender and/or race (Clarke *et al.*, 2009; Lachman *et al.*, 2007). Still others have found no association at all (Glatt *et al.*, 2007; Mayer & Hollt, 2006: Saxon *et al.*, 2005). The picture remains opaque. To date, there does not appear to be any conclusive evidence that reliably links a particular gene to opioid dependence in humans (Meyer & Hollt, 2006). This may not be that surprising, as genetic effects on opioid metabolism theoretically might affect any of the processes involved in metabolising opioids, including absorption, distribution, metabolism and excretion (Kosarac *et al.*, 2009).

It is questionable how much any of this matters clinically when compared to the impact of psychosocial factors. Whether there are, or are not, genetic influences is not of any particularly great clinical or epidemiological significance for the life of the heroin user. Addiction may very well occur at the intersection of genes and environment, as posited by some (Tyrfingsson *et al.*, 2010). It is likely, however, that the genetic influences will be polygenic, with many genes weakly correlated with risk. Environmental factors appear to me to be far more salient. The person must, first and foremost, be exposed to the substance in question which, as we have seen, is significantly more likely to occur in disadvantaged communities and families. The strong association with childhood abuse and neglect, again far more prominent in disadvantaged families, also indicates the importance of environmental and psychological factors in the development of opioid dependence.

2.5 Childhood sexual and physical abuse

General population studies indicate that those with substance use disorders are far more likely to have a history of childhood abuse (Conroy *et al.*, 2009; Molnar *et al.*, 2001). Importantly, predictors of childhood abuse include parental substance abuse, social disadvantage and parental psychopathology, which is almost a redescription of all we have discussed to date on the childhoods of heroin users (Fergusson & Lynskey, 1995, 1997; Knutson *et al.*, 2004). The high rates of parental substance use problems are of particular concern for the possibility of child abuse, given the known links between substance abuse, disinhibition and violence referred to earlier (Athanasiadus, 1999; Darke, 2010; Goldstein, 1985; Phillips *et al.*, 2007). Given the frequently dysfunctional family backgrounds of heroin users, and the fact that heroin use is such an extremely dangerous life 'choice' to make, we would expect abuse to figure prominently in the childhoods of heroin users. We would be correct. Table 2.2 presents the childhood abuse histories of samples of opioid users, and of larger samples of substance users that include heroin users. As can be seen, a history of traumatic childhood abuse is common, indeed the norm.

There are different forms that abuse may take. Firstly, let us examine sexual abuse, which includes penetrative and non-penetrative abuse. As we can see from Table 2.2, the proportions of heroin users who experienced childhood sexual abuse are extraordinarily high, independent of any other forms of abuse that they may have experienced. Studies repeatedly report from a third to more than half of heroin users have experienced childhood sexual abuse. These figures, however, conceal a marked gender difference in exposure to sexual abuse. Female heroin users are substantially more likely than their male counterparts to have experienced childhood sexual abuse, and to have experienced it more frequently. Indeed, an inspection of Table 2.2 indicates that female rates are typically double or more those of males (which are high in themselves). A typical example of this discrepancy is seen in Conroy *et al.* (2009), where three-quarters of female heroin users were sexually abused as children, compared to a third of males. Clinicians dealing with heroin users are thus presented with a population amongst whom sexual abuse histories are common and, indeed, present in the majority of females. The average age that such abuse commences is extremely young, in the order of 8–12 years, and multiple incidents occur in approximately half of those abused (Braitstein *et al.*, 2003; Conroy *et al.*, 2009; Farrugia *et al.*, in press; Gilbert *et al.*, 1997; Ompad *et al.*, 2005).

Child abuse is not restricted to sexual abuse, but also includes non-sexual physical abuse (Table 2.2). As noted above, rates of alcohol and other drug dependence are high amongst the parents of opioid users, and such dependence is associated with a higher risk of familial violence (Fergusson & Lynskey, 1997; Knutson *et al.*, 2004). This risk is seen in the rates of childhood physical abuse amongst heroin users (Table 2.2). Rates of childhood physical abuse are comparable to, or indeed higher than, those of sexual abuse. Under the term physical abuse, we include behaviours such as beating, slapping, choking and burning. One major difference between these two forms of abuse, however, is the absence of a consistent gender effect. Unlike sexual abuse, males and females appear equally likely to be victims of childhood physical abuse. Again, clinicians dealing with heroin users will typically find that at least half have been physically abused as children.

Finally, we must not ignore emotional abuse and physical neglect, although this is not studied as frequently as sexual and physical abuse (Table 2.2). Emotional abuse includes such things as verbal abuse, frequent shaming and embarrassment and constantly being ignored or told you are worthless. Clearly such abuse will also be likely to have ramifications for normal psychological development. Where reported, rates of childhood emotional abuse are typically 50% or higher. Again, where reported, rates of physical neglect of users as children (e.g. not fed properly, not properly clothed, not given appropriate medical care) are substantial. The overall pattern of abuse and neglect seen in the childhoods of heroin users is corroborated by the fact that large proportions of users were removed from their parents during childhood by child welfare agencies (Deykin & Buka, 1994; Rossow & Lauritzen, 2001; Wu *et al.*, 2010).

The picture of extensive abuse that we have built is one that has been poignantly termed '*shattered childhood*' by Rossow & Lauritzen (2001). We must bear in mind that the different forms of abuse are not mutually exclusive, and large proportions of users suffer multiple types of abuse over their childhoods (Gilbert *et al.*, 1997; Heffernan *et al.*, 2000; Ouimette *et al.*, 2000; Rosen *et al.*, 2002; Rossow & Lauritzen, 2001; Sansone *et al.*, 2009). Given the risk factors for abuse seen amongst their social and parental backgrounds, we would expect these figures to be far in excess of population rates. Such is indeed the case. Rates of abuse and neglect amongst opioid users are far higher than those seen in the general population and matched control groups (Conroy *et al.*, 2009; Heffernan *et al.*, 2000; Ompad *et al.*, 2005; Westermeyer *et al.*, 2001; Wu *et al.*, 2010). Heffernan *et al.* (2000), for example, reported a three-fold increase in the risk of heroin use independently associated with a history of child abuse. As we will see in later chapters, these high levels of violence continue into adulthood, with the same gender imbalance in sexual assault being maintained (Clark *et al.*, 2001; Cottler *et al.*, 1992; Darke *et al.*, 2010e; Hien *et al.*, 2000; Mills *et al.*, 2005). Physical assault is a particular problem for drug users, and by the time the person is around 30, the experience of lifetime violent physical assault amongst both genders is close to universal (Darke *et al.*, 2010e).

So, amongst heroin users, the rates of all forms of childhood abuse are extremely high, and far higher than rates amongst non-users. How much does this matter? Very much indeed. Childhood abuse is associated with higher risks for substance dependence, major depression, dysthymia, PTSD, self-harm and suicide (Darke *et al.*, 2010d; Fergusson & Lynkey 1995; Maloney *et al.*, 2010; Roy, 2009; Wines *et al.*, 2004). Abuse may also lead to involvement in further abusive relationships as an adult (Gilbert *et al.*, 1997). The *extent* of abuse also matters, with more extensive histories predicting subsequent suicidal ideation and attempts (Rossow & Lauritzen, 2001). Amongst injecting drug users (IDU), a history of sexual abuse is associated with an earlier onset of injecting, which is a marker for more severe problems and a poorer long-term prognosis (Ompad *et al.*, 2005).

In later chapters we will examine the incredible chronicity of heroin dependence, and the fact that many, perhaps the majority, never 'mature out' of addiction. When we look at the rates of parental pathology and substance abuse, and the extent of abuse, this should come as no surprise. Our typical heroin user is likely to have been severely traumatised as a child. While self-medication as a hypothesis has been in and out of favour over the years, the high levels of abuse amongst heroin users appears more than a passing coincidence. Opioids are effective physical and psychological pain-killers. Childhood abuse appears to be a major part of the path to dependence, and is particularly relevant to the genesis of female heroin use careers (Plotzker *et al.*, 2007). It is worth noting that female opiate users who attempt suicide do so on average 4–6 years before their male counterparts. Unlike males, this typically occurs *prior* to the commencement of heroin use (Darke & Ross, 2001; Maloney *et al.*, 2009). It not unreasonable to suspect the role of childhood abuse in this pattern of suicidality. We must also note the inter-generational implications of this cycle. The children of heroin users will likely be faced with similar circumstances and risks as their parents before them.

Before moving on to examine the childhood psychopathology of heroin users, brief comment must be made here on resilience. It is not the case that every child who is exposed to abuse will develop severe psychopathology or substance use disorders (Fergus & Zimmerman, 2005; Luthar *et al.*, 2000; Masten & Obradovic, 2006). Some children will overcome the negative effects of risk exposure, although the factors underlying such resilience are not well delineated to date. Despite this, child abuse is a grave assault upon the person, and clearly increases the risk of drug dependence as well as child and adult psychopathology, as discussed in the next section.

2.6   Childhood psychopathology of the heroin user

As we have seen, heroin users carry many risk factors for the development of psychopathology. Parental psychopathology and substance abuse are common and, as we have seen, various forms of childhood abuse are prevalent. Given the *'shattered childhoods'* of so many users, we would be entitled to expect high rates of adult psychopathology amongst this population. This, of course, is exactly what we find (Brienza *et al.*, 2000; Cacciola *et al.*, 2001; Darke & Ross, 1997; Kidorf *et al.*, 2004; Maloney *et al.*, 2010; Teesson *et al.*, 2005).

Whilst adult psychopathology rates are high, many of these disorders or their precursors first manifest during childhood (Ahmadi *et al.*, 2003; Darke *et al.*, 2003c; Hahesey *et al.*, 2002; Lynskey & Fergusson, 1995; Ompad *et al.*, 2005; Pugatch *et al.*, 2001; Rossow & Lauritzen, 2001; Wilens *et al.*, 2002). Given the childhood circumstances described above, this will come as no great surprise. Rossow & Lauritzen (2001), for instance, reported that half their sample had experienced psychiatric problems prior to the age of 16. Similarly, Pugatch *et al.* (2001) reported that one in four adolescent heroin users had psychiatric histories, with females more than twice as likely to have such a history. Moreover, childhood diagnoses frequently precede the onset of substance use and dependence (Hahesey *et al.*, 2002). Importantly, a childhood psychiatric diagnosis is associated with more extensive polysubstance use and an earlier age of drug use initiation (Pugatch *et al.*, 2001). These associations remain important to the adult user, with more extensive dependent polydrug use still being associated with more extensive psychiatric diagnoses (Darke & Ross, 1997).

As with adult pathology, rates of childhood pathology amongst heroin users are far higher than the general population. In part, this is a reflection of the inter-generational transfer of pathology discussed briefly above. At a general level, the children of those with substance abuse and/or psychopathology are more likely to develop mental health problems and substance dependence than the children of controls (Luthar *et al.*, 1993; Nunes *et al.*, 1998; Ohannessian *et al.*, 2004; Wilens *et al.*, 2002). More specifically, the children of opiate users have higher rates of childhood? than matched controls or, indeed, the children of alcoholics (Nunes *et al.*, 1998; Wilens *et al.*, 2002). The latter finding is particularly instructive, as it gives an idea of the level of dysfunction that such children must experience. Furthermore, children with anxiety or depressive symptoms are more likely to begin substance use at an earlier age, and are more likely to develop substance use problems (Cicchetti & Rogosch, 1999; Costello *et al.*, 1999; Henry *et al.*, 1993; Loeber *et al.*, 1999).

Two disorders deserve separate mention: post traumatic stress disorder (PTSD) and conduct disorder (CD). PTSD is a severe anxiety disorder that can develop after exposure to events that result in psychological trauma (APA, 2000). The triggering events involve threats of death, or threats to physical, sexual or psychological integrity, that overwhelm the individual's ability to cope. This is a diagnosis of particular relevance to us, given the high rates of childhood abuse experienced by this population. Amongst adult heroin users, lifetime diagnoses of PTSD are in the order of half or more, compared with a population prevalence of 8% (Mills *et al.*, 2005). Given what we have seen in the childhoods of users (*prior* to the violence associated with adult drug dependence) this appears to be a major pathway to addiction amongst heroin users. As we noted earlier, the cycle is likely to repeat in the children of the heroin users we are discussing in this book.

As adults, antisocial personality disorder (ASPD) is one of the most common diagnoses amongst heroin users (Darke *et al.*, 2004c). While the diagnosis of ASPD is bedevilled with theoretical problems (as we will see in Chapter 5), the mandatory predecessor to this adult diagnosis is CD, which, by definition, must have developed prior to the age of 15 (APA, 2000). An adult may not receive the diagnosis of ASPD unless they satisfy criteria for CD. The advantage of CD as a prognostic diagnosis is that it is less likely than adult ASPD to be confounded by behaviours generated by drug dependence. Rates of CD are extremely high amongst heroin users, as are histories of juvenile arrest (Darke *et al.*, 2003c; Hser *et al.*, 2007a; Wilens *et al.*, 2002). The diagnosis is important, as children who engage in antisocial behaviours are far more likely to develop substance use problems (Cicchetti & Rogosch, 1999; Fergusson *et al.*, 1993; Lynskey & Fergusson, 1995). The earlier, more varied and more serious a child's antisocial behaviours, the more likely they continue into adulthood, including substance abuse (Costello *et al.*, 1999; Lynskey & Fergusson, 1995). It is tempting to conclude that heroin users are 'born bad' and their later use of drugs merely reflects these antisocial tendencies. We must bear in mind, however, the rates of childhood abuse experienced by this population, and the modelling of children on the behaviours of substance dependent parents.

2.7 Summary

There is a far higher likelihood that a heroin user will have come from a disadvantaged background than a more privileged one. As we have seen, this also tends to be associated with what is termed 'shattered childhood'. Of course, this is not true of every user. Some obviously will come from wealthier backgrounds, and/or may well have had perfectly decent parents who did not have serious psychopathology, use drugs or abuse their children. The reverse is also true: not everyone who has these experiences will develop heroin dependence The data, however, indicate that poverty and shattered childhood are strongly predictive of heroin dependence later in life. Given the extent of the abuse in the backgrounds of heroin users described in this chapter, this is not surprising. The move to heroin use, however, still lies some years in the future for our heroin user. Typically, this journey commences at a young age with other, less dangerous drugs. We will explore the initial steps into substance use in the next chapter.

Key points: Summary of parents and childhood

- Social disadvantage is associated with poorer physical and mental health, including higher rates of substance dependence.
- Children of parents with substance abuse disorders are significantly more likely to develop substance use disorders themselves.
- Rates of substance abuse, psychopathology and conflict amongst the parents of heroin users are high.
- Research from twin, adoption and family studies suggest that there may be a genetic component that increases the likelihood of opioid dependence.
- It has been suggested that genetic variations in the mu opioid receptors may influence how opioids are metabolised. To date, however, there is no conclusive evidence that has reliably linked any particular gene to the development of opioid dependence in humans.
- People with substance use disorders are more likely than others to have a history of childhood abuse.
- A third to half of heroin users experience childhood sexual abuse.
- Female heroin users are substantially more likely to have experienced child-hood sexual abuse, and to have experienced it more frequently.
- Childhood abuse has been associated with higher risks for substance depend-ence, major depression, dysthymia, PTSD, self-harm and suicide.
- Rates of childhood physical abuse are comparable to those for sexual abuse. One major difference between these two forms of abuse is the absence of a consistent gender effect for physical abuse.
- Rates of childhood psychopathology amongst heroin users are high.

3

Early teenage years: the onset of substance use

3.1 Introduction

We have seen that the typical heroin user is likely to come from a background that contained a great many risk factors for substance use. We have also seen that initiation into heroin use carries with it an extremely high risk of developing dependence on the drug. It is extremely unlikely, however, that the first experience of intoxication will be with heroin. Typically, a range of licit and illicit psychoactive substances will have been experimented with prior to commencing heroin use. In this chapter we will examine the entry into substance use of the future heroin user, an event that usually occurs in the early teenage years. Before we look more specifically at the substance use histories of heroin users, we will first examine 'gateway theory' as a possible explanation for the development and progression of substance use and dependence (Kandel, 2002).

3.2 The gateway hypothesis

The gateway hypothesis arose in the mid-1970s and is, essentially, a description of the developmental trajectories of substance use derived from observations of sequencing patterns in the initiation of substance use (Kandel, 1975, 2002). The concept of sequencing, however, goes back at least to the 1930s, with what was termed 'Stepping Stone Theory' (cf. Kandel, 2002). Gateway theory (also known as the 'gateway pattern' and the 'gateway effect') postulates that there are developmental stages, and sequences, of involvement in psychoactive drugs. A progressive, and hierarchical, sequence of stages in drug use is posited. Thus, the use of drugs that are earlier in the sequence (i.e. lower in the progression hierarchy) predicts progression to the use of drugs later in the sequence (i.e. higher in the hierarchy). Four developmental stages were identified. Stage 1 is the initiation into licit drug use, predominantly by means of alcohol and cigarettes. Stage 2 involves the initiation of cannabis use, typically the first of the illicits to be used. Stage 3, which is of particular relevance to this book, involves initiation into the use of other illicit 'hard' drugs, such as the psychostimulants and heroin. Finally, Stage 4 involves the use of prescribed psychoactive pharmaceuticals, such as opioid analgesics, although this is considered by Kandel and colleagues to be the weakest link in the sequencing pattern (Kandel *et al.*, 1992). Essentially, the hypothesis is that the use of less deleterious drugs substantially increases the risk of using more dangerous 'hard' drugs, with their higher levels of risks for dependence, health problems and criminal involvement. It is important to note that gateway theory does *not* assume that drugs used in earlier stages will be disregarded after progression to later stages. Rather, there typically will be an accretion of drug classes, leading to the patterns of polydrug use so often seen amongst heroin users and other 'Stage 3' drug users. One implication of this probabilistic progression is that the likelihood of use of later sequenced drugs might be reduced by preventing the initiation of earlier stages. The 'gateway' to the next stage is, effectively, narrowed.

It is important to note that this sequence is *not* viewed as an inexorable progression. Clearly, that would be absurd. Not all who use alcohol go on to use cannabis, for instance, and the same can be said for each stage progression. Rather, it is a probabilistic sequence, in which the initiation of drug use in one stage of the sequence increases the probability of initiating drugs from the next stage. Drugs at one stage thus provide the *gateway* to the next. Cannabis, in particular, is often termed a gateway drug, as it is seen as the portal to other illicit (and more dangerous) drug use (Kandel, 2002; Morral *et al.*, 2002; van Ours, 2003). It is this probabilistic approach that distinguishes gateway theory from earlier incarnations, such as Stepping Stone Theory, which saw stage progressions as inexorable, at least for the progression from cannabis to heroin (Kandel, 2002). Even though postulating a probabilistic sequence, we can still view the relationships between stages as causally linked, in that initiation into one stage predicts an increased probability of progression to the next stage (Fergusson *et al.*, 2006; Van Gundy & Rebellon, 2010).

The mechanisms that could underlie such a sequence are still not entirely clear. At the biochemical level, it has been argued that the use of cannabis may alter the neurochemistry of the brain, increasing responsiveness to other illicit substances (Ellgren *et al.*, 2007). More specifically, it has been asserted, on the basis of animal studies, that cannabis alters the neural opioid receptor system, which affects hedonic processing, thus increasing the risk of heroin dependence (Ellgren *et al.*, 2007). Alternative explanations of the gateway sequence concern the individual, or their social setting (Fergusson *et al.*, 2006). At the individual level, one possibility is that, when experimenting with cannabis, the person learns that it has pleasurable effects, and low rates of adverse effects. This learning experience is then generalised to experimentation with other illicit drugs. At the social level, there will be, almost by definition, differences between the social associations of cannabis users and non-users. Cannabis users are far more likely to be in contact with drug users and dealers, and a milieu that includes the use and normalisation of other illicit drugs. In this conceptualisation, the cannabis gateway is thus viewed as an introduction to a drug using culture. It increases the availability of drugs to the individual and, thus, the likelihood of their being used.

3.2.1 *The evidence for gateway theory*

Regardless of the theoretical explanation for gateway sequencing, there has been a range of evidence supporting the existence of such a progression (Fergusson *et al.*, 2006; Fleming *et al.*, 1998; Golub & Johnson 2002; Kandel *et al.*, 1992; Kandel & Yamaguchi 1999; Oh *et al.*, 1998). Support for the sequencing trajectory has come from longitudinal cohort studies, and retrospective modelling of cross-sectional data. One of the broader findings that supports gateway theory is that the risk for initiation into illicit drug use is mostly over by the age of 20 (Chen & Kandel 1995; Degenhardt *et al.*, 2000). Presumably, if the adolescent developmental trajectory through licit to illicits has not been engaged by this age, it is unlikely that the person will commence illicit drug use of any sort. In particular, it is unlikely that cannabis use will commence after the age of 20, which suggests that other illicit drug use is also unlikely.

The temporal primacy of licit drugs in the gateway sequence is well documented (Fleming *et al.*, 1998; Golub & Johnson, 2002; Kandel & Yamaguchi 1999, 2002; Kandel *et al.*, 1992; Oh *et al.*, 1998). Typical of such research, Kandel *et al.* (1992) reported that only 5% of cannabis users had commenced cannabis use prior to cigarettes or alcohol, and less than 1% of 'other illicit' drug users had commenced illicit drug use without such prior exposure. Typically, cigarette use precedes that of alcohol. Age of onset data from national studies, and those of established illicit drug users, also support this stage of the sequence (Golub & Johnson, 2002;

Kandel & Yamaguchi, 2002). In one such US national household study, onset ages were: cigarettes (14.3yrs), alcohol (16.2yrs), cannabis (16.6yrs), heroin (20.1yrs), cocaine (20.2yrs) (Kandel & Yamaguchi, 2002).

A great deal of research has centred on cannabis as the gateway to further illicit drug use (Fergusson *et al.*, 2006; Fergusson & Horwood, 2000; Golub & Johnson, 2002; Kandel, 1984; Kandel *et al.*, 1992; Kandel & Yamaguchi, 2002). Most who use cannabis will *not* progress to the use of 'harder drugs', such as cocaine or heroin. A large number of studies, however, have reported that it is rare for the user of 'hard' drugs not to have initiated cannabis use prior to the other illicits. Typically, less than 10% of illicit drug users did not commence illicit use with cannabis. Fergusson *et al.* (2006), for instance, reported that 98% of those with illicit drug use histories commenced cannabis use prior to, or in the same year as, other illicits. Similarly, Kandel (1984) reported that only 7% of youth who had never used cannabis reported other illicit drug use. Consistent with these figures, Fergusson & Horwood (2000) estimated that weekly cannabis users were 59 times more likely to use other illicit substances.

The final stage, the progression to the use of prescribed psychoactive substances, is less well documented (Kandel *et al.*, 1992). Kandel *et al.* (1992) remarked that this fourth stage of development was a weaker member of the sequence, with substantially more sequence violations than between earlier stages. Importantly, since the 1990s there have been marked changes in the prescription opioid market. As we have noted, there is considerable concern about the abuse of oxycodone (Carise *et al.*, 2007; Cicero *et al.*, 2005; Darke *et al.*, 2011; Paulozzi, 2006). The question now being asked is whether oxycodone may act as a gateway drug to heroin, and there appears to be some evidence to support this (Grau *et al.*, 2007).

3.2.2 Alternative interpretations of drug initiation sequencing

Not all authors agree with gateway theory, nor are all data consistent with it (Agrawal *et al.*, 2004; Breslau *et al.*, 2004; Degenhardt *et al.*, 2009a, 2010; Morral *et al.*, 2002; Wells & McGee, 2008). The arguments about gateway theory relate to cultural specificity, temporal specificity and alternate explanations that involve a rejection of the entire concept of a 'gateway' drug.

One of the problems in extrapolating gateway sequences to international use patterns is that the overwhelming majority of research has been conducted in cultures where tobacco, alcohol and cannabis use are highly prevalent (Degenhardt *et al.*, 2010). The question is thus whether the gateway sequence is seen in cultures in which these substances are *not* widely used. Recent cross-cultural comparisons from the World Health Organization's World Mental Health Survey suggest that the gateway sequence is culturally dependent (Degenhardt *et al.*, 2010). Higher rates of order violations in the use of licit and illicit drugs are seen in countries where the prevalence of alcohol and tobacco is lower than in the cultures traditionally studied. In South Africa, for instance, cannabis use levels are moderate, and rates of alcohol and cannabis use the lowest of the 17 countries studied. It also has the highest levels of sequencing violations, with one in seven South African cannabis users *never* having used licit substances prior to cannabis. Similarly, there is poorer adherence to the Stage 2–Stage 3 progression in countries where the prevalence of cannabis use is low (e.g. Japan, Nigeria, South Africa). In Japan, for instance, the prevalence of other illicit drug use (e.g. psychostimulants) is in *excess* of that of cannabis, the reverse of what we would expect from the gateway sequence.

In both of these stage progressions, sequencing appears related to the background prevalence of the drugs, rather than to any inherent characteristics of the substances themselves. Overall, the association between drug initiation differed across countries, and was associated to the prevalence of the 'gateway' drug in question. These findings suggest that the traditional gateway sequence may be an artefact of the cultures in which they were conducted, cultures with a high prevalence of alcohol, tobacco and cannabis use. It may well describe onset patterns in such cultures. Rather than any innate properties of drugs that determine sequencing, however, it would appear that access and cultural attitudes are crucial.

Temporal specificity is also problematic. Drug markets are dynamic, and there are marked cohort effects in substance use patterns across generations (Breslau *et al.*, 2004; Degenhardt *et al.*, 2009a; Weiss *et al.*, 1988; Wells & McGee, 2008). Both Wells & McGee (2008) and Degenhardt *et al.* (2009a) reported that sequencing violations were more common amongst recent cohorts, in which the prevalence of substance use is higher than in previous cohorts. Importantly, these studies were based upon data from New Zealand and the USA, where the prevalence of both licit precursors and cannabis are high, and where the gateway sequencing pattern is strong. Sequencing thus does not appear to be set in stone, but is temporally sensitive. The issue may be considered more broadly. A far stronger association between tobacco smoking and psychiatric morbidity is now being observed, as the prevalence of smoking has declined in many countries (Breslau *et al.*, 2004). Similarly, the reverse is observed for the association between cocaine and psychopathology, which weakened as the use of cocaine became more widespread and normative amongst some sections of the community (Weiss *et al.*, 1988). Finally, as noted previously, the rapid increase over the course of the last decade in the prescribing of oxycodone has meant that this may be the *first* opioid used, and may lead to the use of heroin (Grau *et al.*, 2007).

It would appear that sequencing is far from an inviolate progression. The observed primary sequence will depend upon both the country, and time, in which it was observed. There are further problems with the traditional concept of gateway drugs. Associations between stages should be consistent. Thus, reductions in the use of a gateway drug, such as cannabis, should be associated with reduced rates of dependence upon other illicits. Violations in sequencing order, however, appear to have no relation to the risk of dependence (Degenhardt *et al.*, 2009a; Wells & McGee, 2008).

If gateway sequences are not universal, then how do we conceptualise the early trajectory of the dependent drug user? At a theoretical level, it would appear that reductionist approaches that emphasise the inherent effects of substances upon the brain face many problems (Ellgren *et al.*, 2007; Schenk, 2002). As we have seen, there is nothing fixed about sequencing orders. Indeed, most who use cannabis do *not* go on to use, or become dependent upon, heroin. It is difficult to see how cannabis-induced neurochemical alterations could be causally associated with the later use of the wide range of substances used by Stage 3 users, such as the psychostimulants, hallucinogens and heroin, which operate through entirely different receptor systems. Furthermore, as we have seen, there are an overwhelming number of well-documented psychosocial risk factors for progression to the use of harder drugs.

Finally, independent of specificity there is, in my opinion, a major theoretical problem in the entire concept of Stage 3 (i.e. other illicit drug use). The drugs in this stage are defined by their illegal status, and by not being cannabis. The stage thus includes drugs as disparate in harm and dependence potential as MDMA, methamphetamine, hallucinogens and heroin. Pharmacologically, these drugs have little in common. To collate them in a common stage appears to miss the importance of their differences, and of their sequelae. A move from cannabis to occasional MDMA use, a drug with low dependence liability and mortality risk, is a very different matter from a move to heroin. Furthermore, transitions between routes of administration are also crucial in determining substance use progression. Methamphetamine use, for instance, often precedes heroin use. A person who is injecting methamphetamine, however, is far more likely to inject heroin if it becomes available to them than if they are inhaling or smoking the drug (Darke *et al.*, 1999b). The transition from non-parenteral use to injecting is a crucial stage in drug use careers, and appears to lie outside the gateway stages, which focuses on substances *per se*.

I consider our best hope for explanation to reside in the psychosocial domain, not in neurobiology. Rather than posit gateway drugs, it has been proposed that sequencing can be more parsimoniously explained by a common factor model, in which common causal factors underlie all substance use (Agrawal *et al.*, 2004; Degenhardt *et al.*, 2009a; Morral *et al.*, 2002; van Ours, 2003). In such a model, the entire concept of a 'gateway' is discounted. Rather, some individuals are, for whatever reasons, willing to try psychoactive substances, and the 'gateway' drugs are merely the ones that are more readily available at an earlier age than are other drugs. There are thus common factors that underlie drug use *per se*, with psychopathology in particular having been noted (Degenhardt *et al.*, 2009a). The high levels of abuse, neglect and psychopathology seen amongst heroin users, explored in the previous chapter, are clearly relevant here. Cannabis is usually the most available illicit drug, and exposure to the black market (in which harder drugs are likely to be available) will likely result in what *appears* to be a gateway sequence. Rather than a sequence, the early onset of substance use *per se* will increase the likelihood of other drug use, as all use is being driven by the same underlying factors. An advantage of this concept is that the problems of cultural and temporal specificity seen in gateway theory are avoided. There *is no* formal sequence, merely those most likely to occur in the particular place and time, amongst those most socially and psychologically at the highest risk of use.

3.3   Trends in the age of substance use initiation

As noted above, drug markets are dynamic and there are marked differences between successive cohorts in patterns of drug use and initiation. Several major trends that have implications for drug use trajectories have emerged since World War II. Firstly rates of illicit substance use have increased across each successive cohort (Degenhardt *et al.*, 2000, 2008; Johnson & Gerstein, 1998, 2000; Mills *et al.*, 2004; Perkonigg *et al.*, 2006; Roxburgh *et al.*, 2010; Wells & McGee, 2008). Whilst initiation into the traditional licit substances has remained relatively stable, the extent of illicit drug use across cohorts is substantially different. As alluded to earlier, the higher prevalence and normalisation of illicit substance use has implications for the dynamics and sequencing of drug use initiation. Whatever the explanation for sequencing, there is no doubt that in recent cohorts there is greatly increased exposure to illicit drugs, and the opportunities to use them. The move into illicit drug use is many magnitudes greater amongst young people at the time of writing than it was even 30 or 40 years ago.

The second major trend of note is that the age of initiation to both licit and illicit drugs has declined (Degenhardt *et al.*, 2000; Johnson & Gerstein, 1998, 2000; Lofwall *et al.*, 2005; Mills *et al.*, 2004; Perkonigg *et al.*, 2006; Roxburgh *et al.*, 2010; Wells *et al.*, 2006). In addition to being more likely to initiate illicit drug use, each successive cohort has commenced the use of both illicits and licits at an earlier age than the preceding cohort. Such a trend has serious clinical implications. It is well established that an earlier age of onset for substance use is associated with higher levels of dependence, and swifter and more severe problem development (Degenhardt *et al.*, 2008; Fergusson & Horwood, 1997; Mills *et al.*, 2004; Perkonigg *et al.*, 2006; Roxburgh *et al.*, 2010). Earlier onset users tend to meet 'career milestones', such as dependence and first treatment entry, at earlier ages than later onset users. Again, whatever the explanation for sequencing, all theories would concur that such a trend increases the probability of the wider use of *all* illicit drugs. Heavier use of a substance increases the probability of going on to use other substances. For instance, the heavier the use of, and dependence upon, cannabis, the more likely are other drugs to be used. Younger cohorts are commencing use younger, are thus more likely to develop dependence and thus be at risk for more extensive polydrug use.

3.4 Early licit substance use among heroin users

Whether we accept the tenets of gateway theory, or alternative explanations of sequencing patterns, we would expect widespread exposure to other drugs amongst people who have progressed to the dependent use of heroin. We would not be wrong, as we will discuss below. Typically, heroin users experience their first intoxication with a psychoactive substance (excluding tobacco) at around the age of 13–14 years old (Abelson *et al.*, 2006; Bennett & Higgins, 1999; Darke *et al.*, 2010c,e; Darke & Ross, 2001; Golub & Johnson 2002; Ompad *et al.*, 2005). We will now briefly examine the main drugs that are taken up by the typical heroin user in their teens.

3.4.1 Tobacco

Studies of adult heroin users consistently show tobacco smoking to be almost universal (McCool & Richter 2003; Ross *et al.*, 2005). Amongst any sample of heroin users, whether in treatment or not, we would expect to find that at least 95% smoke cigarettes, even amongst older users aged in their 50s (Ross *et al.*, 2005). This is an excellent example of the accretion of substance use referred to above in the adult polydrug user, which we will fully examine in Chapter 5. The typical age of initiation into tobacco use for a heroin user is usually around 12–14 years (Abelson *et al.*, 2006; Bailey *et al.*, 1994; Golub & Johnson 2002; Kandel & Yamaguchi, 2002; San *et al.*, 1991). There are a couple of points to note about this pattern. Firstly, it means that heroin users are exposed to the harmful effects of tobacco smoking, including pulmonary and cardiac disease, over the course of decades, as they maintain their smoking. While this may not be of especial importance for the nascent drug user in their early teens, it will be recalled that nicotine is the only psychoactive substance to have a greater dependence liability than heroin, and that early onset of any drug is associated with heavier dependence. There are serious implications for health in middle age from decades of smoking (in addition to all the other exigencies of the heroin lifestyle). As we shall see in Chapter 7, there is a strong pattern of accelerated ageing amongst heroin users, including far poorer cardiovascular and pulmonary functioning than would be expected for age and gender. At least part of this may be due to the early onset of smoking, and its sheer chronicity among this group.

A second important implication of this early onset of smoking is that the person has made the transition to psychoactive drug use, even if it is a 'soft' drug. Furthermore, the act of learning to smoke and inhale may make for an easier transition into the use of cannabis. It should also be noted that many cannabis smokers mix cannabis with tobacco when smoking cannabis.

3.4.2 Alcohol

Alcohol use and dependence will become one of the most important clinical aspects for heroin users across their lifetime. The lifetime use of alcohol by heroin users is close to universal, and use typically commences around the age of 13–14 years, generally slightly after the initiation of tobacco use (Abelson *et al.*, 2006; Bailey *et al.*, 1994; Carpentier *et al.*, 2009; Darke *et al.*, 1998; Golub & Johnson 2002; Ompad *et al.*, 2005; Pugatch *et al.*, 2001). As we have seen, there does not appear to be an inviolable order for alcohol and other drugs. Given its widespread availability in many societies, however, alcohol often constitutes the first intoxicating substance used by heroin users.

While many of the complications of alcohol use, such as hepatic and cardiovascular disease, will only manifest in later years, there are immediate potential consequences for adolescents that are of great clinical concern. It has long been known that alcohol is neurotoxic, and that debilitating amnestic disorders such Korsakoff's Psychosis may result from heavy use and poor nutrition (APA, 2000). There is emerging evidence, however, from both human and animal research that adolescents may be far more vulnerable to the effects of alcohol than adults (Clark *et al.*, 2008; Lubman *et al.*, 2007; Medina *et al.*, 2007; National Institute on Alcohol Abuse and Alcoholism, 2004/5; Nixon & McLean, 2010). At the neurological level, there is emerging evidence that alcohol use in adolescents is associated with reduced hippocampal volumes and white matter abnormalities in the corpus callosum. This is a period of extensive neuromaturation, and it would appear that alcohol negatively affects the normal maturational process, with likely cognitive sequelae such as memory deficits (Lubman *et al.*, 2007). Of course, neuromaturation is not the only form of maturation occurring in the adolescent. This is a period of great hormonal and physical development. Again, human and animal studies indicate that adolescents are at heightened vulnerability to alcohol across a range of organ systems. Adolescents appear more prone to liver disease, reduced levels of oestrogen in girls and testosterone in boys and lowered bone density (National Institute on Alcohol Abuse and Alcoholism, 2004/5). It should be noted that, apart from a special vulnerability, adolescents may be further at risk due to *reduced* vulnerability to the sedative effects of alcohol and motor discoordination, which may lead to higher levels of binge drinking and harm (White *et al.*, 2002).

There are thus serious and immediate sequelae from early alcohol use that may have long-term negative effects on normal maturation. In later years, however, alcohol will come to form a stable component of the polydrug use patterns for many heroin users, and large proportions will develop dependence on the drug (Brugal *et al.*, 2002; Darke & Ross, 1997; Hubbard *et al.*, 1997; Kidorf *et al.*, 2004; Quan *et al.*, 2007). This is of serious concern for a population that already carries a high risk for mortality and morbidity, as alcohol dependence is in itself a risk factor for early mortality, due to the extensive range of disease it engenders (Harris & Barrclough, 1997). The high rates of hepatitis C (HCV) infection amongst heroin users also has implications, as alcohol use will exacerbate the damage to the liver. Finally, alcohol is a major contributor to what are termed 'heroin' overdoses, as we shall see in later chapters (cf. Darke *et al.*, 2007a).

3.5 Early illicit substance use among heroin users

3.5.1 Cannabis

Lifetime cannabis use in samples of heroin users is typically in excess of 90% (Ross *et al.*, 2005). Moreover, rates of both use and dependence amongst mature users remain extremely high. The average onset of cannabis use by heroin users typically occurs in the period between 14 and 16 years of age (Abelson *et al.*, 2006; Carpentier *et al.*, 2009; Dinwiddie *et al.*, 1996; Hser *et al.*, 2007a; Lofwall *et al.*, 2005; Ompad *et al.*, 2005; Pugatch *et al.*, 2001). It needs to be reiterated that cannabis may, in some cultures, be the first substance used *per se*, depending on the national prevalence of use and availability (Degenhardt *et al.*, 2010). Even in western cultures where the traditional sequencing pattern is prevalent, cannabis use may precede that of alcohol (Abelson *et al.*, 2006; Golub & Johnson 2002). Overall, the early to mid-teens are a period of extensive drug initiation amongst those who will later become heroin users. Rather than the sequence *per se* being of interest here, it is the developing involvement in substance use that is of clinical importance. As noted above, the fact that most will be smoking tobacco may substantially 'lower the bar' for smoking other substances.

As with other drugs, many of the problems associated with cannabis use will only manifest in later life (Hall *et al.*, 1999). There are, however, more proximal associations with early onset cannabis use, such as that demonstrated by heroin users, that may dramatically affect later life (Horwood *et al.*, 2010; Rothman & Stephens, 2006). Perhaps of greatest importance is the association of early onset cannabis use with poor educational attainment (Fergusson *et al.*, 1993; Horwood *et al.*, 2010; Lynskey & Hall 2000; Van Ours & Williams, 2009). This is unlikely to be a statistical artefact. Even after controlling for potential confounders, early onset, heavy cannabis use is related to higher rates of school drop-out, and lower rates of secondary completion and of tertiary education (Horwood *et al.*, 2010). Intuitively, if one is frequently getting 'stoned', it is likely that school performance will decline. Drugs will also increase in their importance to the new user as time progresses. This is of direct relevance to our heroin user. As we will see in Chapter 5, mature heroin users typically have low levels of educational achievement. This will, by necessity, impact upon employment opportunities in later life, and most heroin users will experience long periods of unemployment. It is likely that the downward social mobility seen amongst many heroin users has its genesis in early onset adolescent substance use.

Finally, much has been spoken of in the media in recent years on cannabis psychosis. In particular, there has been considerable public concern that cannabis use may engender schizophrenia. Despite the media hysteria surrounding the issue, the evidence for such an association is scant (Degenhardt *et al.*, 2007; Degenhardt & Hall, 2002; Rothman & Stephens, 2006). There is some evidence from longitudinal studies that cannabis use increases the risk of developing psychosis (Rothman & Stephens, 2006; van Os *et al.*, 2002; Zammit *et al.*, 2002). The effect size, however, is small, and there are serious problems in determining onset orders (Degenhardt *et al.*, 2007). Moreover, large-scale studies report that symptoms of psychosis do *not* predict cannabis use (Degenhardt *et al.*, 2007). Finally we must bear in mind that the epidemiology of cannabis use and schizophrenia mitigate against attributing any strong association between cannabis and psychosis. As we have noted earlier in this chapter, rates of cannabis use have increased dramatically over the preceding 50 years across the world. Over the same period, however, rates of schizophrenia have remained stable or *declined* (Degenhardt *et al.*, 2003). If cannabis is a substantial contributor to the development of psychosis, we should have seen a substantial rise of rates of schizophrenia that parallels the increased prevalence of cannabis use. No such pattern has emerged.

The generally accepted picture, based upon research, is that cannabis may precipitate schizophrenia in those who were genetically vulnerable to the disease, and precipitate relapse to psychosis in those already affected by the disorder. Overall, however, it appears unlikely that cannabis causes psychosis in those who are not vulnerable to it (Degenhardt *et al.*, 2007; Degenhardt & Hall, 2002; Rothman & Stephens, 2006). Certainly, there is no evidence for elevated rates of psychosis amongst mature heroin users, despite their having typically smoked cannabis for decades.

3.5.2 *Psychostimulants*

As with cannabis, lifetime exposure amongst heroin users to psychostimulants is close to universal (Darke *et al.*, 1999b; Gossop *et al.*, 2002a). At first blush, this may sound rather odd, as the psychostimulants are, as the name indicates, stimulants ('uppers') whilst heroin is a soporific, CNS depressant ('downer'). Between a third and half of mature heroin users will have recently used either cocaine or methamphetamine, and a substantial proportion will meet criteria for dependence on these drugs (Abelson *et al.*, 2006; Bargagli *et al.*, 2006; Cacciola *et al.*, 2001; Darke & Ross,

1997; DeMaria *et al.*, 2000; Flynn *et al.*, 2003; Gossop *et al.*, 2000; Miller *et al.*, 2007; Ross *et al.*, 2005; Williamson *et al.*, 2007).

The type of psychostimulant that predominates is, to a degree, dependent upon the location of the individual, and the cyclic drug patterns that see epidemics recur across decades. In North America and Europe, cocaine dominates the psychostimulant market, although there have been waves of methamphetamine epidemics in the USA. Marked increases have been noted in recent years in methamphetamine use around the Pacific Rim, including western North America, south-east Asia and Oceania (UNOCD, 2009). The average onset age for methamphetamine amongst heroin users is typically in the late teens, between 17 and 19 years old, with cocaine initiation also around this time or slightly later (Abelson *et al.*, 2006; Bailey *et al.*, 1994; Carpentier *et al.*, 2009; Dinwiddie *et al.*, 1996; Hser *et al.*, 2007a; Lofwall *et al.*, 2005; Pugatch *et al.*, 2001; San *et al.*, 1991).

The use of psychostimulants has been related to the transition to heroin use by some authors (Darke *et al.*, 1999b; Inciardi & Harrison, 1998). This may be due to several factors. Firstly, the injection of psychostimulants is a strong predictor of later heroin injecting (Darke *et al.*, 1999b). If the late teens psychostimulant user is injecting the drug, the transition to injecting another substance is relatively minor, compared to the transition to injecting *per se*. Secondly, there is evidence that heavy psychostimulant use may lead to heroin use as a means of taking the 'edge' off the effects of the psychostimulants, such as anxiety and insomnia (Inciardi & Harrison, 1998). A psychostimulant epidemic such as the US crack epidemic of the 1990s may, counter-intuitively, engender a new generation of heroin users.

As we shall discuss in some detail later, there are a great many reasons to be concerned about long-term psychostimulant use, with particular issues relating to heroin users. There are reasons, however, to be concerned also about the acute sequelae of psychostimulant use. Firstly, there is the danger of an acute, schizophreniform psychosis, involving symptoms such as paranoid delusions and hallucinations. Even in the absence of psychosis, clinically significant psychotic symptoms are common amongst psychostimulant users (McKetin *et al.*, 2006).

The second major problem is that psychostimulants are cardiotoxic, and place substantial demands upon the cardiovascular system (Darke *et al.*, 2008a; Karch 2009; Kaye *et al.*, 2007). While there are long-term sequelae that will be discussed later, sudden acute aortic dissection and coronary vasospasm may occur in young people with no underlying coronary artery disease. Indeed, chest pains and other cardiovascular symptoms are the most common presenting symptoms in emergency departments relating to acute psychostimulant intoxication. There is also a substantially increased risk of stroke. Crucially, there is no known dose–response between psychostimulant use cardiovascular accidents, which may occur on any occasion of use.

3.6 Early sexual activity

Finally, we must mention the initiation into sexual activity by the developing heroin user. The early teens is a time of great transition for all youth, but particularly for the heroin user. As we have seen, for a heroin user the transition into substance use, and initial intoxication, typically occurs in the very early teens. This early transition to what could be termed 'adult behaviours' is also seen in sexuality. There is an extensive literature linking early onset substance use and sexual initiation in the pre-teens or very early teens (Garofalo *et al.*, 1998; Plotzker *et al.*, 2007; Santelli *et al.*, 2004; Shrier *et al.*, 2001; Stueve & O'Donnell, 2005; Westermeyer *et al.*, 2001). Thus, earlier onset ages of tobacco, alcohol and cannabis use are associated with onset of sexual behaviours in the 11–14-year-old range, more sexual partners and a higher risk of premarital pregnancy. This is of particular relevance for the nascent heroin user since, as we have seen above, there is a dominant pattern of early onset drug use that typically precedes initiation into heroin. The early onset of Stage 3 illicits is particularly associated with early sexuality (Garofalo *et al.*, 1998; Shrier *et al.*, 2001; Stueve & O'Donnell, 2005). Such research also indicates that early substance use not only predicts early sexuality, but higher levels of sexual risk. The picture is one of premature and precocious development. It is not only drug use that appears to commence around puberty for the developing heroin user.

In discussing emergent sexuality, we must bear in mind that we are speaking here of *consensual* sex. As we saw in Chapter 2, rates of childhood abuse amongst heroin users are high, particularly amongst females. Not surprisingly, given the traumatic severity of such events, abuse has strong associations with later sexual development and behaviours. Drug users who were sexually abused as children exhibit higher sexual risk-taking in later life, including higher rates of unprotected sex, more sexual partners, a higher probability of prostitution and higher rates of sexually transmitted diseases (Arriola *et al.*, 2005; Braistein *et al.*, 2003; Dube *et al.*, 2005; Plotzker *et al.*,

2007; Westermeyer *et al.*, 2001). Furthermore, as we shall see in Chapter 5, large proportions of heroin users, particularly females, engage in sex work to support their heroin use. We should note here that PTSD and depression also predict early sexual initiation. Such associations give pause for thought, given the rates of childhood abuse seen amongst heroin users. Such abuse would appear to be a major risk factor for the early emergence of both drug use *and* sexual behaviours. The fact that so much risk is undertaken at such a young age, and by so many, cannot be a coincidence.

3.7 Summary

Whether one adheres to gateway theory or common factor models as explanatory mechanisms, for the heroin user, the early teens are a time of deepening licit and illicit drug involvement. They are also a period in which many users begin consensual sexual activity. Overall, there appears to be a pattern of precocious development in the substance use and sexual spheres. One could argue that it is too much too young. Our soon to be heroin user stands on the edge of the transition to heroin use, and all that this implies. We will explore this transition, and its immediate consequences, in the next chapter.

Key points: Summary of early teenage years: the onset of substance use

- Gateway theory postulates that there is a progressive, hierarchical sequence of stages of drug initiation: (i) licit drug use, (ii) cannabis use, (iii) other illicit drug use, (iv) prescription pharmaceutical use.
- Support for the sequencing trajectory has come from longitudinal cohort studies, and retrospective modelling of cross-sectional data.
- Gateway sequencing appears to be subject to both cultural and temporal specificity, with different sequences observed across different countries and times.
- Rather than posit gateway drugs, it has been proposed that sequencing can be more parsimoniously explained by a common factor model, in which a common causal factor underlies all substance use.
- The drugs in Stage 3 are defined by their illegal status, and by not being cannabis. The stage thus includes drugs that are widely disparate in harm and dependence potential.
- Rates of illicit substance use have increased across each successive cohort, and each successive cohort commences illicits and licits drug use at an earlier age.
- Heroin users typically are first intoxicated with a psychoactive substance (excluding tobacco) at around the age of 13–14 years old.
- There is emerging evidence that adolescents are more vulnerable to the effects of alcohol than adults.
- Early onset cannabis use is associated with academic underachievement.
- There are acute risks of psychosis and cardiovascular accidents associated with psychostimulant use.
- As with substance use, there is early initiation of sexual activity amongst heroin users, with first consensual sex occurring in the early teens.

4

The mid to late teens: commencing heroin use

4.1 Introduction

We come to the point of heroin initiation, moving on to using the most dangerous drug of all. As we have seen, from around puberty, a wide range of drugs typically will have been used. Whether one subscribes to gateway theory or common cause models, the path to heroin almost always lies through involvement with other drugs. Heroin is, with good reason, a drug that is viewed as dangerous and carries a high stigma, as is clearly reflected in the epidemiology of its use relative to other drugs. It is very unlikely that a drug with such stigma would be the one that people choose to commence drug use. Rather, we would expect involvement in a range of more 'acceptable' drugs to precede heroin use. In this chapter we will examine the age of onset for heroin use, routes of administration and the harms associated with the early heroin use career.

4.2 Initiating heroin use

4.2.1 Age of initiation

The mean ages for heroin initiation from major studies are presented in Table 4.1. As we can see, there is remarkable consistency between these studies, conducted across 4 continents and 14 countries. The average age of onset in these studies is just under 20 years, within a remarkably narrow range. The lowest onset age was 14.5 years (Abelson *et al.*, 2006), reported amongst a group of 'early onset' users, and the oldest was 25.9 (Chen *et al.*, 2010). It is clear that the late teens and early 20s pose by far the greatest risk for initiating heroin use. When we consider the journey into heroin use, one thing that stands out is the brevity of the time between first use of any substance and that of first heroin use. Over the space of just 8 years in a

Table 4.1. Onset ages for heroin use, regular use and injecting drug use

Study	Country	Age of first heroin use	Age of first regular use/ dependence	Age of first injected drugs
Abelson *et al.* (2006)	Australia	15.9 (early onset 14.5, late 17.3)	–	17.4 (early onset 15.3, late 19.4)
Anglin *et al.* (1986)	USA	18.5	20.3	–
Bailey *et al.* (1994)	USA	18.1	19.6	–
Balakireva & Grund (2006)	Ukraine	–	–	17.7
Bargagli *et al.* (2001)	Italy	20.0	–	–
Bargagli *et al.* (2006)	Italy	19.6	–	–
Bauer *et al.* (2008)	Austria	18.4	–	–
Bennett & Higgins (1999)	UK	–	–	20.4
Best *et al.* (2002)	UK	–	–	20.9
Boeri *et al.* (2008)	USA	19.0 (early onset 19.0, late 40.0)	–	–
Capenter *et al.* (1998)	USA	21.1	–	–
Chen *et al.* (2010)	Taiwan	25.9	–	–
Chiang *et al.* (2006)	Taiwan	18.6	–	–
Cooncool *et al.* (1979)	USA	18.2	–	–
Dean *et al.* (2004)	Australia	22.3	–	–
Darke *et al.* (1996a)	Australia	–	–	18.8
Darke *et al.* (1996b)	Australia	19.3	20.9	–
Darke *et al.* (1998)	Australia	18.6	–	–
Darke *et al.* (1999b)	Australia	19.1	–	18.4
Darke *et al.* (2007c)	Australia	18.0	–	–
Darke & Ross (2001)	Australia	20.0	21.3	–
Degenhardt *et al.* (2000)	Australia	Born 1970–1974:20.0 1975–1979:18.0	–	–
Degenhardt *et al.* (2008)	Australia	–	–	<25 yrs: 15.0, 25–34: 17.0, >34: 19.0
Digiusto *et al.* (2004)	Australia	20.4	–	–
Gossop *et al.* (1992)	UK	19.2	–	–
Gossop *et al.* (1996)	UK	20.6	–	–
Gossop *et al.* (1998)	UK	20.3	–	–

Table 4.1. (*contd.*)

Study	Country	Age of first heroin use	Age of first regular use/ dependence	Age of first injected drugs
Griffiths *et al.* (1994)	UK	19.0	–	–
Haarstrup & Jepson (1988)	Denmark	–	17.0	–
Haasen *et al.* (2007)	Germany	22.5	–	–
Hartnoll *et al.* (1980)	UK	18.0	–	–
Hser *et al.* (2007a)	USA	17.9	–	–
Inciardi & Harrison (1998)	USA	21.0	–	–
Kandel & Yamaguchi (2002)	USA	20.1	–	–
Kalyoncu *et al.* (2007)	Turkey	17.8	–	–
Kelly *et al.* (2004)	USA	23.9	–	–
Khantzian & Treece (1985)	USA	20.0	–	–
Lofwall *et al.* (2005)	USA	Aged 25–34: 19.3, 50–66:	– –	– 24.2
Luty (2003)	UK	21.2	24.1	–
Lynskey & Hall (1998)	Australia	Born 1940–1949: 20.5 1970–1979: 16.5	–	–
Man *et al.* (2002)	UK	19.8	–	21.8
McGlothlin & Anglin (1981)	USA	–	19.6	–
McGregor *et al.* (1998)	Australia	19.9	–	–
Mills *et al.* (2004)	Australia	16.8	17.3	< 25 yrs
Neaigus *et al.* (2001)	USA	22.4	–	–
Neaigus *et al.* (2006)	USA	22.3	–	–
Noble *et al.* (2002)	UK	20.0	–	–
Nurco *et al.* (1981)	USA	18.2	–	–
O'Driscoll *et al.* (2001)	USA	–	–	20.7
Ochoa *et al.* (2001)	USA	–	–	18.0
Perez-Jimanez & Robert (1997)	Spain	20.7	–	–
Powis *et al.* (1996)	UK	19.0	–	–
Powis *et al.* (1999)	–	–	–	20.0

Table 4.1. (*contd.*)

Study	Country	Age of first heroin use	Age of first regular use/ dependence	Age of first injected drugs
Pugatch *et al.* (2001)	USA	18.2	–	–
Robertson *et al.* (1993)	UK	20.4	–	–
Ross *et al.* (2005)	Australia	19.6	–	–
Ross & Darke (2000)	Australia	19.4	–	–
Rounsaville *et al.* (1985)	USA	20.3	–	–
Rutherford *et al.* (1994)	USA	23.2	–	–
San *et al.* (1991)	Spain	19.6	–	–
Sanchez-Carbonell *et al.* (1988)	Spain	19.0	–	–
Sanchez-Carbonell & Seus (2000)	Spain	18.7	–	–
Seal *et al.* (2001)	USA	–	–	20.0
Sergeev *et al.* (2003)	Russia	18.0	–	18.0
Sheehan *et al.* (1988)	UK	20.4	–	–
Smyth *et al.* (2000)	Ireland	19.7	–	–
Strang *et al.* (1997)	UK	19.3	–	–
Strang *et al.* (1999a)	UK	18.7	–	–
Strang *et al.* (1999b)	UK	–	–	20.1 (heroin 20.5)
Surratt *et al.* (2004)	USA	23.4	–	–
Vaillant (1973)	USA	–	23.0	–
van Ameijden *et al.* (1994)	Netherlands	–	20.3	–
Warner-Smith *et al.* (2002)	Australia	20.3	21.7	–

young life (even less in more recent cohorts), the average user moved from cigarettes and alcohol, through many other drugs, to using the most dangerous drug of all. Of course, we have seen that, for far too many users, the groundwork for this was laid in childhood, years before drug use commenced. It needs to be stated here again, however, that the progression to heroin use is *not* inevitable.

Interestingly, there does not appear to be a noticeable gender difference in onset ages (Balakireva & Grund, 2006; Bargagli *et al.*, 2006; Degenhardt *et al.*, 2008; Kandel & Yamaguchi, 2002). As noted earlier, it is one of the most robust features of the international literature that males constitute around two-thirds of heroin users. While females may be less likely to engage in illicit drug use, and heroin use in particular, those who do, appear to exhibit the same trajectories in their adolescence as their male counterparts. This is consistent with the work of Van Etten & Anthony (1999), which we discussed earlier, who reported that, while males were twice as likely to have had an opportunity to use heroin, there was no gender difference in the *likelihood* of using once an opportunity did arise.

As discussed in Chapter 3, recent years have seen a decline in the age of initiation for licit and illicit drugs (Degenhardt *et al.*, 2000; Lofwall *et al.*, 2005; Mills *et al.*, 2004; Roxburgh *et al.*, 2008; Wells *et al.*, 2009). Both gateway and common factor theory would predict that such a movement towards earlier onset would be reflected in declines in the age of heroin initiation. In the case of gateway theory, this would occur because gateway drugs are being used earlier, and such exposure increases the odds of the earlier use of drugs from later in the sequence. Similarly, common factor models would predict an earlier onset of heroin use due to earlier involvement in polydrug use. Whatever the correct interpretation, the decline in onset ages *is* reflected in earlier heroin involvement (Degenhardt *et al.*, 2000; Lofwall *et al.*, 2005; Lynskey & Hall, 1998; Mills *et al.*, 2004). Degenhardt *et al.* (2000) reported a linear decline across 30 years, from 33 years old at onset for the 1945–1949 Australian birth cohort, to 18 years old for the 1975–1979 cohort. Similarly, Lofwall *et al.* (2005) noted that the mean onset age amongst younger US heroin users (aged 25–34) was 5 years less than that that of their older counterparts (aged over 50). As we noted earlier, such a trend has serious clinical implications, as an earlier age of onset predicts higher levels of dependence and more severe drug-related problems (Fergusson & Horwood, 1997; Grant & Dawson, 1998; Mills *et al.*, 2004; Perkonigg *et al.*, 2006; Roxburgh *et al.*, 2010). Consistent with this, long-term 'enduring' addicts will typically commence their heroin use at an earlier age than 'early quitters', who exhibit a far briefer trajectory (Bailey *et al.*, 1994; Hser *et al.*, 2007a).

In Chapter 3, we noted that the abuse liability of heroin is second only to that of nicotine (Nutt *et al.*, 2007). This is amply demonstrated in the astonishingly brief time-lag between initial use and the development of regular, dependent use patterns. In the studies where this lag has been reported (Table 4.1), the average time between initiation and dependent use was only around 18 months (Anglin *et al.*, 1986; Bailey *et al.*, 1994; Darke *et al.*, 1996b; Darke & Ross, 2001; Luty, 2003; Mills *et al.*, 2004; Warner-Smith *et al.*, 2002). Thus, within 2 years of initiation, there is a very high likelihood that a regular, dependent use pattern will have emerged, with all that this implies for the welfare of the individual.

4.3 Routes of heroin administration

The two main routes of heroin administration are injecting or smoking ('chasing'). In the case of the latter, a more accurate term is inhalation, as we shall see below. Of course, a powder such as heroin may also be inhaled nasally ('snorted, sniffed'), as cocaine often is, or simply swallowed. We must also bear in mind that even oral pharmaceutical opioids, such as methadone syrup, may be injected by dependent users. Overwhelmingly, however, heroin is either injected or smoked, the two routes upon which we shall now focus.

4.3.1 Injection

In most industrialised nations the use of heroin has traditionally been by injection. As we noted in Chapter 1, the twin developments of the hypodermic syringe and heroin in the nineteenth century resulted in injecting becoming the dominant route of administration across the ensuing years. Heroin users will typically inject the drug intravenously. This is not necessarily the case, however, as some users simply inject into muscle tissue ('skin popping'). It was for this reason that the nomenclature was amended from '*intravenous* drug users' to '*injecting* drug users', a matter of great indifference to those thus described. The initial injection will typically be in the cubital fossa (the crook of the arm), although a wider range of injecting sites typically emerges across the use career, as we will see in later chapters (Darke *et al.*, 2001b; Hoda *et al.*, 2008).

The average onset age of injecting drug use from the studies presented in Table 4.1 is around 19 years, again within a very narrow range. Readers will note that this is slightly younger than that of heroin onset from the same table. This reflects the fact that, as alluded to in Chapter 3, heroin may not be the first drug injected. We have already seen that a heroin user will almost certainly have used a wide range of drugs prior to heroin, including injectable substances such as methamphetamine and cocaine. While many heroin users do commence injecting with heroin, not surprisingly a large proportion begin their injecting careers with other drugs, most commonly the psychostimulants (Abelson *et al.*, 2006; Balakireva & Grund, 2006; Crofts *et al.*, 1996; Darke *et al.*, 1999b; Roberts *et al.*, 2010). We should not assume, however, that, once the injection of heroin occurs, the injecting career has reached its logical conclusion. Even if other substances were not injected previously, once the transition to injecting has occurred, other injectables will probably be used in this manner. Similarly, as dependence develops, and contact with treatment services increases, we may also see the injection of pharmaceutical products, such as methadone, buprenorphine and the benzodiazepines (Darke *et al.*, 1997, 2002b; Guichard *et al.*, 2003; Humeniuk *et al.*, 2003; Jenkinson *et al.*, 2005; Kintz, 2001; Ross *et al.*, 1997; Vidal-Trecan *et al.*, 2003).

The move to injecting is a major landmark in the life of an IDU. Who exactly is it that inducts the new user? To inject drugs into a vein is a process that must be learnt. After all, medical staff must be trained in it. From the images given in the media, one could be forgiven for thinking that the inductor is some nefarious drug dealer, lurking around to initiate the unwary. The truth is far more prosaic: induction by dealers is extremely rare (Abelson *et al.*, 2006; Balakireva & Grund, 2006; Crofts *et al.*, 1996; Doherty *et al.*, 2000; Powis *et al.*, 1996; Roy *et al.*, 2002; Vidal-Trecan *et al.*, 2002). It is true that it is unusual to commence injecting use alone, or without guidance. The person must learn how to prepare the drug for injection, how to locate a vein, and how to inject into that vein. Missing the vein, or hitting an artery, can have serious consequences. The initial injection most commonly occurs in a home, with established IDU friends and/or sexual partners present. It is they who guide and initiate the new IDU, prepare the drugs and, in most cases, inject the person (Abselson *et al.* 2006; Balakireva & Grund, 2006; Crofts *et al.*, 1996; Doherty *et al.*, 2000; Powis *et al.*, 1996; Roy *et al.*, 2002; Vidal-Trecan *et al.*, 2002). There do, however, appear to be some gender differences in who inducts the new IDU, with women more likely to be initiated by a sexual partner, and men by a friend.

4.3.2 Smoking

While injection has been the 'traditional' route of heroin administration in industrialised nations, the latter part of the twentieth century saw significant changes in use patterns. While heroin smoking has been reported in Asia since the 1920s, large-scale non-parenteral heroin use is a relatively recent phenomenon in western countries (Strang *et al.*, 1997). Since the 1990s, there have been substantial increases in the use of heroin by smoking in the United

Kingdom (Strang *et al.*, 1997, 1999a), Europe (Perez-Jimenez & Robert, 1997; Smyth *et al.*, 2000; van Ameijdan *et al.*, 1994), the United States (Carpenter *et al.*, 1998; Fuller *et al.*, 2002; Neaigus *et al.*, 2001, 2006) and Australia (Darke *et al.*, 2004a, 2005b, 2008b; Swift *et al.*, 1999).

The widespread non-parenteral use of heroin first appeared in the Netherlands in the 1970s, in the UK and Europe in the 1980s and in the USA, Australia and India from the 1990s. The rise of heroin smoking in the Netherlands is an excellent illustration of how cultures may change their patterns of drug use. In the Netherlands, the Surinamese migrant community was the spur for a major change in administration routes. Many Surinamese migrated to the Netherlands in the late 1970s, when the former colony was granted independence (Strang *et al.*, 1997). Two important events occurred. Firstly, much of the low level heroin distribution came under the control of young members of this community. Secondly, needle use was frowned upon in this culture, and these heroin users smoked the drug. The contact between this group of distributors and Dutch users saw the spread of heroin smoking to the wider Dutch heroin using community. The practice subsequently spread throughout Europe from this central node (Strang *et al.*, 1997).

Strictly speaking, we are not usually speaking about smoking as such. Of course, some users literally do smoke the heroin in a cigarette or cannabis bong. Most commonly, however, we are referring to the inhalation of heroin vapours. The drug is placed upon aluminium foil, or some other metal object, which is then heated. The user then inhales the vapourised heroin through a tube or rolled up banknote. The term 'chasing the dragon' or simply 'chasing' is commonly used, referring to chasing the vapour plume as the heated heroin moves around the foil. One of the major factors enabling the rise in the proportion of heroin users who are happy to smoke the drug has been the increase in the availability of brown heroin from south-west Asia. As we saw earlier, this is a free base that is easily smoked (EMCDDA, 2010). In contrast, south-east Asian heroin is typically a white powder, and more suited to injection. When brown heroin started appearing in major European drug markets, the proportion of users who smoked was directly related to the proportion of the market taken up by brown heroin (de la Fuente *et al.*, 1996).

This trend has generated a great deal of clinical interest, as heroin smoking is associated with reduced risk for both overdose and viral infection (Carpenter *et al.*, 1998; Darke & Ross, 2000; Gossop *et al.*, 1996; Swift *et al.*, 1999). We shall discuss this in more detail later in this chapter. We should not leave this section, however, without commenting on the long-term trajectories of heroin smokers. As we shall see in later chapters, while there is reduced risk for overdose and viral infection, there are serious long-term harms for the mature heroin smoker. It should not be seen as a 'safe' route by which to use heroin. There is no safe route. The drug itself carries a high degree of risk, regardless of how it is administered.

4.3.3   Transitions between routes of heroin administration

We should not assume that the route of heroin administration of a user is immutable. There is, of course, a great deal of consistency in routes of administration. Users are not prone to change their predominant route of administration at whim, and many will stay with their predominant route throughout their entire use career. The move from one route to the exclusive (or near exclusive) administration by another means is termed a *transition*. Studies generally set a mark for a transition of a month's use by a different primary route (Darke *et al.*, 2008b; Griffiths *et al.*, 1994). An IDU who occasionally smokes heroin when the situation demands it (e.g. where no needles are available) would *not* be classified as having made a transition to smoking. They would have to move to smoking as their regular, primary route of administration for us to consider that a transition has occurred. There has to be a degree of consistency in the behaviour.

By definition, a transition may be between any two routes of administration. Overwhelmingly, however, the most common transition is from smoking (chasing) to injecting (Darke *et al.*, 2008b; Fuller *et al.*, 2002; Griffiths *et al.*, 1994; Neaigus *et al.* 2001, 2006; Perez-Limenz & Robert, 1997; Pugatch *et al.*, 2001; Strang *et al.*, 1997, 1999a; van Ameijden *et al.*, 1994). In the initial research from the UK, 45% of smokers had made a transition to injecting (Griffiths *et al.*, 1994), with a similar figure seen amongst Spanish users (Perez-Limenz & Robert, 1997). Amongst the Australian Treatment Outcome Study (ATOS) cohort, a third of baseline smokers injected over the course of 3 years and 10% made a transition to injecting (Darke *et al.*, 2008b). None had injected a drug prior to this. These figures are close to those seen over 5 years amongst Dutch heroin users (van Ameijden *et al.*, 1994), while amongst US smokers a fifth moved to injecting over 7 years (Neaigus *et al.*, 2001). Griffiths *et al.* (1994) calculated the risk of making the transition to injecting to be 10% per annum. In contrast, transitions from injecting to smoking in these studies are far rarer. In ATOS, for example, only 10% of injectors smoked heroin at all across 3 years, and only 2% made a transition to smoking (Darke *et al.*, 2008b). Overall, the data suggest that injecting is the most stable route of administration, nasal inhalation ('snorting') the least durable, with smoking lying somewhere in-between (Strang *et al.*, 1997).

It is crucial to note that the average number of life transitions in these studies is *one*. That is, once a transition has occurred, the person tends to stay with the new route. Overwhelmingly, this consists of the move to injecting, from which it is very rare to make a return. The 'rush' from injecting, as the bolus crosses the blood–brain barrier, is a powerful reinforcer. The move to a route that involves smaller, repeated doses does not appear to carry a great deal of appeal for the established injector.

There are thus three routes into injecting heroin use, which we may think of as injecting trajectories. The first is simply to initiate injecting with heroin. The second is an established injector of other drugs, typically the psychostimulants, who makes the transition to injecting heroin. The third trajectory is a transition from non-injecting heroin use to injection. It should be clear to readers by now that route of administration is a crucial factor in the development of drug dependence, and of opioid dependence in particular. Rather than focus on the drug *per se*, we must remember that the route of administration is a major factor in transitions between primary drug classes.

4.4   The harms of early stage heroin use

As we shall see in subsequent chapters, a great many of the more serious harms associated with heroin use will only manifest after some years of use. There are, however, harms that apply to the early career use, and that presage the troubles to come.

The obvious new risk is overdose. While both fatal and non-fatal overdose occur with other drugs, the risk is far higher for heroin than for any other drug (Darke *et al.*, 2007a). Indeed, as we will see, overdose is one of the two major killers of heroin users (Darke *et al.*, 2007a). While overdose will play a major role in the life of most users, it is one that typically occurs later in their use career, after the development of dependence. Of course, overdoses do occur amongst new users. They are, however, very unusual. The time between initiation into heroin use and first non-fatal overdose is approximately 2 to 3 years (Darke *et al.*, 1996b; Gossop *et al.*, 1996). It is not the new user who is at greatest risk, but the established, regular user. The demographics of fatalities confirm this, with the mean age of cases being in the early 30s, and very few cases under the age of 20 (Darke *et al.*, 2007a). Once the person commences heroin use, there is a constant risk of overdose, a risk that appears to increase across time. The route of administration is of major importance, with injecting associated with a substantially higher risk. Smokers can, and do, overdose, as do 'sniffers'. Their risk, however, is substantially lower, as injecting delivers a morphine bolus to the brain, while in smoking the dose is titrated across a number of use episodes.

The second risk for the new heroin user is blood-borne disease. Strictly speaking, this is a risk associated with injection rather than heroin. The major viral infections of concern are HCV, hepatitis B (HBV) and human immuno-deficiency virus (HIV). The risk for infection is related to receptive needle sharing (using a needle and syringe after another person has used it) for all of these viruses, and from sexual transmission for both HIV and HBV. If the new user is an established IDU, then the risk merely continues. It may be exacer-bated, however, since heroin is associated with regular, and more sustained, injecting than the psychostimulants, and we know that more frequent injecting is a strong marker for infection. The other infection of concern is infective endocarditis, also transmitted through needle sharing, which we shall discuss in the next chapter. Finally, we must keep in mind that injectors, even if they *never* share needles, do regular vascular damage by the very act of injecting. This is something that is often overlooked in the (understandable) focus on reducing viral transmission rates. Even the new injector is doing damage, however, that will accumulate over time. Of course, we must bear in mind that the heroin smoker will, by definition, not be exposed to these disease risks. There are other disease risks, however, to which they are uniquely prone, as we shall discuss in the next chapter.

There are also immediate social implications for the new user. We have seen the high dependence liability of heroin, and the relatively short time-lag between initiation and dependence. This has immediate implications for the new user in obtaining the money to support what is a very expensive 'habit', typically well in excess of what could be supported by a wage, even if the person was employed. Two possibilities present themselves. Firstly, commit-ting acquisitive property crime or drug dealing to support the habit. As we shall see in the next chapter, most regular heroin users will become deeply involved in crime. Furthermore, the strongest factor that predicts criminal behaviour amongst this group is their level of heroin use (Flynn *et al.*, 2003; Gossop *et al.*, 2000). As use increases so, typically, will crime. Of course, this is not to say that crime may not precede drug use. In many cases it does (Hall *et al.*, 1993; Kaye *et al.*, 1998; Torok *et al.*, in press). Even so, the impact of regular heroin use upon the new heroin user will very likely lead to a substantial increase in criminal activity. This will have serious implications for the new user in terms of arrest, imprisonment and loss of employment opportunities due to having a criminal record. The second means for obtaining funds is sex work, common amongst female users, but which also occurs in a substantial minority of males (Surratt *et al.*, 2004). This exposes the new user to a number of immediate risks, most notably violence and sexually transmitted diseases.

Finally, we saw in Chapter 2 that there is extensive abuse and childhood psychopathology amongst this population. Many users will come to heroin use with pre-existing psychiatric morbidity. Heroin use is, however, an extremely hard life. The exigencies of the lifestyle are likely to exacerbate any existing personal distress, and engender distress in those without pre-existing pathology. Indeed, amongst established users, well over half qualify for a psychiatric diagnosis other than drug dependence.

4.5 Summary

The teenage years have come to a close. Over that period we saw the developing heroin user move from their first experiments in substance use in their early teens, through to the initiation of use of the drug with the highest risks for morbidity and mortality. There is also a high risk that they may have transitioned to more dangerous routes of administration. Our user now stands at the commencement of their heroin use career, if not of their drug career *per se*. The new user will now be exposed to a wide range of risks that will dramatically affect their lives. In the next chapter we will examine the patterns of drug use that develop, and the substantial harms that the established user faces.

Key points: Summary of the mid to late teens: commencing heroin use

- The average age of onset for heroin use is around 19–20 years old.
- The age of initiation into heroin use has declined as has that of other illicit drugs.
- The time-lag between heroin initiation and dependent use is approximately 18 months.
- The two main routes of heroin administration are injecting and smoking ('chasing the dragon').
- The average age of first injection is around 19.
- Other drugs are commonly injected prior to the initiation of heroin, most notably the psychostimulants.
- The dominant transition between routes of administration is from smoking to injecting. The reverse is far less common.
- The average number of lifetime transitions is one.
- Commencing heroin use exposes the new user to the risks of overdose, blood-borne viruses, crime and psychological distress.

5

The 20s and 30s: heroin and polydrug use

5.1 Introduction

The years of initiation into drug use are over, and we now find our heroin user in their 20s and 30s. This period can be viewed as the drug career 'prime', both in terms of drug use, and in the increased likelihood of adverse effects. By this stage, the heroin user is firmly entrenched in extensive polydrug use, derived from use established in their teenage years. We will now examine the patterns of polydrug use commonly associated with heroin use, the harms that commonly arise by this stage of the career and the role of polydrug use in exacerbating these harms.

5.2 Heroin use patterns

Now fully enmeshed in the heroin using lifestyle, our heroin user will probably be using heroin on a daily basis (Gossop *et al.*, 1999; Ross *et al.*, 2005). A typical pattern of 2–3 use episodes daily means that heroin is now the centre of life, with the day taken up with obtaining drugs, using them and recovering. Not surprisingly, given the frequency of use, we would expect our heroin user to be showing physical and psychosocial signs and symptoms of the opioid dependence syndrome.

As we have seen, there is a high likelihood that the user may now be injecting. Whilst the cubital fossa (crook of the arm) is the most common initial injection site, and the most common site used generally, it is not the only site used. The use of other sites becomes more common as dependence progresses, and old injection sites become scarred or there is vascular collapse. Alternative sites such as the neck, groin, hands and feet may be used (Darke *et al.*, 2001b; Hoda *et al.*, 2008). Predictors of using other sites include longer injecting careers and more injection-related health problems. As one site wears out other, more dangerous, sites are employed. This pattern of widening injection sites also applies to the use of opioids such as methadone syrup, which may be injected in sites such as the groin (Darke *et al.*, 1996a; Humeniuk *et al.*, 2003).

In examining use patterns, it is important to note that heroin is *not* typically the sole opioid being used. A range of other opioid analgesics may also be present in the suite of substances being used, and a third of primary heroin users typically report the recent use of other opioids (Flynn *et al.*, 2003; Hubbard *et al.*, 1997; Ross *et al.*, 2005). We will recall Stage 4 of gateway theory, the move on to using pharmaceutical products. Dependent heroin users certainly display a tendency for such use patterns. Such drugs include methadone diverted from the treatment setting, codeine preparations and potent analgesics such as oxycodone. As commented upon previously, it should not be assumed that the use of oral opioid preparations is oral. The injection of methadone syrup through large bore needles and 20 ml syringes is well documented, and is a practice associated with substantial harms to the vasculature and a high risk of overdose.

As noted earlier, the pharmaceutical opioid that has received the most attention in recent years is oxycodone, typically prescribed for moderate to severe chronic pain. As we have noted, oxycodone deaths in the USA now exceed heroin or cocaine cases. Such cases comprise two distinct groups: an older group of chronic pain patients (who may have developed an iatrogenic dependence) and IDU who may be injecting the tablets (Carise *et al.*, 2007; Darke *et al.*, 2011). Heroin users are flexible in response to changes in the drug market. In Australia, for instance, there was an increase in oxycodone use by users after the unprecedented reduction in heroin availability that occurred after 2000 (Day *et al.*, 2004). By 2008, a quarter of IDU reported recent oxycodone use, almost all by injection (Stafford *et al.*, 2008).

5.3 Polydrug use patterns

It is rare that an established heroin user will only use opioids. We have noted the initiation into wide-ranging substance use in the teenage years. By this stage, the typical pattern is for heroin use to be nested within a wide range of polydrug use. We would expect our typical user to have used approximately ten different drug classes in their lives, and half a dozen in any one year. Whilst there are negative sequelae associated with individual drugs, the extent of polydrug use *per se*, regardless of the drugs being used, is strongly predictive of a poorer clinical profile (Darke & Ross, 1997; DeMaria *et al.*, 2000). Higher levels of polydrug use consistently predict a higher likelihood of overdose, suicide, psychopathology and poor treatment outcome. We will now examine the drug classes of major clinical significance: alcohol, benzodiazepines and psychostimulants.

5.3.1 Alcohol

Alcohol is the most commonly used drug, other than opioids, by established heroin users (Stapleton & Comiskey, 2010). This is not surprising for two reasons. Firstly, alcohol is by far the most widely available licit drug in most western countries. On the basis of epidemiology alone we would expect many heroin users to drink. Secondly, we have seen that alcohol is a drug that heroin users initiate very early in their drug use career. Finally, there is an affinity in drug type, as alcohol is in the same family of drugs as heroin, being CNS depressants.

Studies consistently report current drinking by heroin users as ranging between a quarter and three-quarters (Bargagli *et al.*, 2006; Best *et al.*, 1999; Brugal *et al.*, 2002; Caputo *et al.*, 2002; Coffin *et al.*, 2007; Stapleton & Cominskey, 2010). Consistent with the broader epidemiology of alcohol use, male users are more likely to use alcohol than their female counter-parts. Not only do the majority of users drink, but large proportions consume on a heavy and frequent basis, with typically a quarter or more drinking to excess daily (Brugal *et al.*, 2002; Caputo *et al.*, 2002; Darke *et al.*, 2006c; Flynn *et al.*, 2003; Quan *et al.*, 2007). Flynn *et al.* (2003) for instance, reported that 42% of clients entering methadone maintenance were drunk on a daily basis. By way of comparison, population surveys show daily alcohol use in major western countries range between 7% and 16% (Australian Institute of Health and Welfare, 2008; Goddard, 2006; Office of Applied Studies, 2006).

Given that their levels of drinking far exceed those of the general popula-tion, we would expect levels of alcohol dependence to be similarly elevated. This is certainly the case, with the lifetime prevalence of alcohol dependence in the order of two-thirds and current dependence between a quarter and half (Cacciola *et al.*, 2001; Darke & Ross, 1997; Hser *et al.*, 1999; Joe *et al.*, 1999; Kidorf *et al.*, 2004; Maloney *et al.*, 2009). In contrast, population estimates of current dependence in some illustrative countries are: United States (1.3%), New Zealand (1.3%) and Australia (1.4%) (Kessler *et al.*, 2005; Teesson *et al.*, in press; Wells *et al.*, 2006). Levels of alcohol dependence, a *secondary* drug for our population, are thus typically many magnitudes higher than amongst the general population.

As we hinted in Chapter 3, for a number of reasons, alcohol is a serious clinical problem for the primary heroin user. Firstly, heavy alcohol use and dependence are independent risk factors for mortality, regardless of heroin use (Harris & Barrclough, 1997). Indeed, alcohol is the most harmful psychoactive substance used by young and middle-aged adults, and is associated with elevated risk for liver disease, cardiovascular disease, cancers, suicide and traumatic accidents (Murray & Lopez, 1997).

The above are risks that the heroin user shares with the broader population. There are, however, risks in alcohol use that are specific to the active heroin user. Firstly, and most importantly, alcohol is a major contributor to what are termed 'heroin' overdoses (Darke *et al.*, 2007a). The combined effects of alcohol and heroin substantially increase the risk of overdose. Secondly, rates of HBV and HCV are in the order of 70% amongst mature heroin users (Hagan *et al.*, 2007). These viruses damage the liver, and may result in hepatic fibrosis, cirrhosis or cancer. The use of alcohol in conjunction with hepatic disease may affect the disease process in the liver, and may possibly increase the risk of overdose due to poor hepatic metabolism (Darke *et al.*, 2006a). Thirdly, alcohol dependence is a known risk factor for suicide, and is present in approximately half of completed suicides (Darke *et al.*, 2009a; Harris & Barrclough, 1997). Whilst this is a general population issue, it has particular salience for heroin users, as suicide is a major cause of death amongst this population. Finally, there is a well-established association between alcohol and violence (Athanasiadus, 1999; Boles & Miotto, 2003). Again, this is a population level issue, but of particular relevance to heroin users, for whom rates of violent assault are extremely high (Darke *et al.*, 2010e).

5.3.2 *Benzodiazepines*

Heroin users have long been known to have a 'taste' for pharmaceutical preparations, consistent with Kandel's Stage 4. The most commonly used pharmaceuticals by heroin users are the benzodiazepines, the drug class that encompasses hypnosedatives and anxiolytics. Like alcohol, these drugs are CNS depressants. Extensive benzodiazepine use amongst heroin users has been documented, and heroin users frequently seek prescriptions for such medications (Bargagli *et al.*, 2006; Darke *et al.*, 2007b, 2010c). Typically, a third to half of heroin users will use benzodiazepines in any one month, with a marked preference shown for quick onset benzodiazepines with high abuse liability (Bargagli *et al.*, 2006; Darke *et al.*, 2010c; DeMaria *et al.*, 2000; Gelkopf *et al.*, 1999; Gossop *et al.*, 2002a; Haasen *et al.*, 2007). Of course, some of this use may be clinically legitimate, for anxiety or sleep problems. A great deal of use, however, is recreational and well in excess of recommended dosage. It should not be assumed that the use of these drugs is exclusively oral. Indeed, given the extent of injecting amongst heroin users, it should not surprise that considerable proportions inject benzodiazepine tablets for a quicker and more powerful effect (Ross *et al.*,1997).

The use of benzodiazepines is consistently associated with a poorer clinical profile, and is a major indicator of increased harm across a wide range of behaviours, including a higher likelihood of heroin overdose, more frequent needle sharing, more extensive polydrug use, poorer physical health, higher levels of psychological distress and a high risk of benzodiazepine dependence (Darke *et al.*, 2010c; Kerr *et al.*, 2007; Ross *et al.*, 1997). Not surprisingly, the injection of benzodiazepines has been associated with even higher levels of psychopathology and injection-related health problems, including vascular morbidity, amputations and mortality (Ross *et al.*, 1997).

The association between benzodiazepine use and elevated levels of harm is undeniable. How are we to understand this relationship? There are two major alternatives. Firstly, benzodiazepine use may simply be a marker for dysfunction, with the more chaotic heroin user more likely to be using these drugs. Alternatively, there may be a direct association between the use of these drugs and a poor clinical profile. Under this scenario, it is the use of the drugs themselves that causes harm, possibly from effects such as disinhibition and amnesia. The latter view appears more cogent. If benzodiazepine is merely a marker for dysfunction, it should consistently predict performance over time. This is not the case. Rather, it is *current* use that predicts *current* harm, suggesting the effects of the drugs themselves matter (Darke *et al.*, 2010c).

5.3.3 Psychostimulants

The drugs discussed to date, licit and illicit, are all in the depressant class. Given that our target population is a group of primary CNS depressant drug users, the use of other drugs from the same broad family would be expected. The use patterns of the mature heroin user, however, extend far beyond depressants. Substantial numbers of primary heroin users also use psychostimulants, which were usually first used in the teens. The two major drugs of relevance here are cocaine and methamphetamine.

Typically, more than half of US heroin users also use cocaine (Cacciola *et al.*, 2000; DeMaria *et al.*, 2000; Flynn *et al.*, 2003; Miller *et al.*, 2007). Similarly, in the UK one in five methadone entrants had recently used crack, and one in ten methamphetamine (Gossop *et al.*, 1998), with comparably high figures reported from other European countries (Bargagli *et al.*, 2006; Haasen *et al.*, 2007; Stenbacka *et al.*, 2007). In Australia, a third of heroin users entering treatment were current methamphetamine users and 40% were using cocaine (Ross *et al.*, 2005; Williamson *et al.*, 2007).

Is psychostimulant use merely another colourful aspect of the mature heroin user's life, with no clinical implications? The data indicate that such use matters a great deal. Firstly, psychostimulant use is associated with more frequent injecting, needle sharing, sexual risk-taking and a higher sero-prevalence of HIV (cf. Darke *et al.*, 2008). Psychostimulants have a shorter half-life than the opioids, resulting in more frequent use and binges, and the patterns of increased risk in all probability relate to this.

Secondly, the regular use of psychostimulants by all routes of administration has been associated with serious psychiatric sequelae, including paranoia, anxiety, depression and excited delirium (APA, 2000). A key clinical difference between the psychostimulants and opioids is that psychostimulant use may induce a paranoid schizophreniform psychosis, with paranoid delusions and hallucinations. Case–control studies have demonstrated that psychostimulant users have higher levels of psychosis compared with users of opioids, benzodiazepines and barbiturates who do not used these drugs (Curran *et al.*, 2004; Farrell *et al.*, 2002). There is also a documented relationship between psychostimulant use and violent offending (Darke *et al.*, 2010e).

Finally, the psychostimulants are distinguishable from the opioids in that they are known to be cardiotoxic, and to place heavy demands upon the cardiovascular system by increasing heart rate and blood pressure (Darke *et al.*, 2008a; Kaye *et al.*, 2007). Two of the most serious sequelae of psychostimulant use are cardiovascular and cerebrovascular complications, both of which occur regardless of route of administration. These will be discussed further in Chapter 8.

5.4   Drug-related problems

As heroin use becomes more regular, and dependence develops, a range of serious drug-related problems emerge. While we have noted that some problems emerge early in the use career, it is the established user who is most at risk. The major problems associated with regular heroin use include overdose, psychiatric and health problems, social deprivation and crime.

5.4.1 Overdose

The most prominent, and dangerous, problem that the established heroin user faces is overdose. Overdose is a result of the CNS depressant effects of opioids leading to a sustained reduction in respiration, and consequent anoxia. As we will see later, overdose is the single biggest killer of heroin users (Chapter 8). As we noted earlier, despite myths to the contrary overdose does not typically occur amongst new heroin users. It is typically only after several years of heroin use that overdoses commence, being associated with higher levels of heroin dependence and more extensive polydrug use.

While overdose is associated in the public mind with death, this most certainly is not the case. It is estimated that the proportion of heroin overdoses that result in death is between 2% and 4% (Darke *et al.*, 2003b). Thus, for every fatal overdose, we can expect 25–50 'near misses'. The prominence of overdose in the life of the regular heroin user is demonstrated by lifetime overdose histories. Studies consistently report that one- to two-thirds of users have overdosed, usually on multiple occasions, with annual rates being in the order of 15%–25% (Backmund *et al.*, 2009; Bargagli *et al.*, 2006; Bradvick *et al.*, 2007; Britton *et al.*, 2010; Darke *et al.*, 2007a,e; Fisher *et al.*, 2004; Kerr *et al.*, 2007; Sergeev *et al.*, 2003; Wines *et al.*, 2007).

Non-fatal overdose is of clinical significance as it is associated with a range of serious sequelae, including pulmonary oedema, bronchopneumonia, rhabdomyolysis ('crush syndrome'), peripheral neuropathy, renal failure, cognitive impairment and traumatic injuries sustained during overdose (Warner-Smith *et al.*, 2001, 2002). Whilst some of these sequelae result from the direct effects of opioids themselves (e.g. pulmonary oedema), others are the physical results of prolonged unconsciousness. Thus, rhabdomyolysis may arise from prolonged pressure on limbs during coma, with resultant renal failure from the lysis of muscle tissue. Prolonged anoxia may result in diffuse organic brain damage with associated cognitive impairment. It must be borne in mind that the responses of heroin users at overdoses is generally poor, due to a fear of police involvement, and prolonged periods of coma and reduced oxygen saturation are common (Baca & Grant, 2007; Bennett & Higgins, 1999; Bradvik *et al.*, 2007; Darke *et al.*, 1996c; Sergeev *et al.*, 2003; Tobin *et al.*, 2005). Given the reluctance to seek help, it is not surprising that survivors often have morbidity resulting from their overdoses.

Overdoses are *not* random events, which is most fortunate as it allows scope for intervention. A number of factors have emerged that strongly predict overdose (Coffin *et al.*, 2007; Cook *et al.*, 1998; Darke *et al.*, 2007a, e; Powis *et al.*, 1999; Seal *et al.*, 2001; Sergeev *et al.*, 2003; Wines *et al.*, 2007). Firstly, a history of overdose strongly predicts future overdoses. Thus, those who overdose are likely to do so again. Secondly, heroin overdoses are associated with more frequent use, and with higher levels of dependence. It is, in all probability, for this reason that overdoses do not typically commence early in the use career. Related to this is the finding that non-fatal overdoses overwhelmingly occur when the person is *not* enrolled in drug treatment, when use is at its peak. Whilst the picture here is one of high heroin tolerance (due to frequent use), there are occasions of reduced tolerance that increase transient overdose risk. In particular, the reinstatement of use after periods of abstinence, such as having been in prison, detoxification or naltrexone maintenance, is associated with a substantially elevated risk (Bradvik *et al.*, 2007; Coffin *et al.*, 2007; Digiusto *et al.*, 2004; Farrell & Marsden, 2007; Kerr *et al.*, 2007; Stewart *et al.*, 2004; Wines *et al.*, 2007).

How heroin is used is also of importance. In particular, injecting is associated with the highest risk for overdose, due to the delivery of a bolus to the brain (Brugal *et al.*, 2002; Carpenter *et al.*, 1998; Darke *et al.*, 2004a, 2005b, 2008b; Milloy *et al.*, 2008; Swift *et al.*, 1999; Yin *et al.*, 2007). Overdoses *do* occur from non-injecting routes of administration, but at far lower rates. Where people use heroin also matters. Street injecting increases the risk, possibly due to a quicker injecting process in order to avoid detection (Darke *et al.*, 2001a; Kerr *et al.*, 2007). Finally, perhaps the most important finding to emerge on overdose risk is that what are termed 'heroin' overdoses typically involve the concomitant consumption of other drugs (Backmund *et al.*, 2009; Bradvik *et al.*, 2007; Coffin *et al.*, 2007; Darke *et al.*, 1996b; Kerr *et al.*, 2007; Sergeev *et al.*, 2003; Yin *et al.*, 2007). The drugs most commonly implicated for increased risk of an overdose are alcohol, benzodiazepines, tricyclic antidepressants and the psychostimulants. Most opioid overdoses (fatal and non-fatal) are, in fact, cases of multiple drug toxicity. This issue will be more fully explored in Chapter 8 when we discuss mortality.

5.4.2 Health

By the time the heroin user has matured into the polydrug using, entrenched user we have been describing, their health will almost certainly have suffered (Neale & Robertson, 2005; Tobin & Latkin, 2003). Much, although certainly not all, of this ill health relates to injection as a route of administration, and to viral transmission through the sharing of injecting equipment.

The related health problem that has had the greatest impact worldwide is HIV infection. The prevalence of HIV among IDU varies considerably by region. A seroprevalence of more than 50% in IDU populations has been reported in many countries, particularly in parts of the United States and southern Europe (Aceijas *et al.*, 2004; Mathers *et al.*, 2008). In contrast, some countries with relatively established IDU populations, such as Australia, have a very low prevalence of HIV (1%–3%) (Mathers *et al.*, 2008). Even within high prevalence countries or cities, rates may vary considerably. Needle sharing is the main vector for HIV infection amongst injecting heroin users and, unfortunately, the sharing of injecting equipment remains a common practice, particularly with sexual partners (Ross *et al.*, 2005). The more frequent the needle sharing, the higher the risk for contracting HIV. Higher levels of dependence (associated with more frequent use) also provide a stronger motivation to inject with shared equipment, as the person is more 'desperate' for the drug.

Whilst certain injecting behaviours are known risk factors for HIV infection, the polydrug use of the heroin user is also related to the likelihood of infection. For instance, people who inject 'speedballs' (heroin and cocaine injected together) are at higher risk of HIV infection than other IDU, due to more frequent needle sharing (Darke *et al.*, 2008a; Doherty *et al.*, 2000). Similarly, benzodiazepines use amongst heroin users is strongly associated with elevated needle risk, due to disinhibition, and/or short-term memory impairment whilst intoxicated (Darke *et al.*, 2010c).

Sexual transmission of HIV is a significant factor for heroin users. In high seroprevalence countries, drug users with a larger number of sexual partners are more likely to be HIV positive (Doherty *et al.*, 2000). As we have mentioned, many heroin users engage in sex work to support their use, which places them at greater risk of contracting HIV.

The other main viral infections that the heroin user is likely to contract are HBV and HCV. As noted above, these are blood-borne viral infections that affect the liver, and may result in cirrhosis or cancer. As with HIV, the predominant mode of transmission of HCV is through injecting drug use. Chronic HCV infection is estimated to occur in three-quarters of infections, and something like 10% of chronic HCV carriers will develop cirrhosis within 20 years, and a fifth by 40 years (Hallinan *et al.*, 2005). It is worthy of note that morphine (the primary metabolite of heroin) appears to enhance HCV viral replication, and inhibits the effectiveness of interferon treatment

(Li *et al.*, 2007). Continued heroin use thus, in and of itself, may contribute to poorer health amongst the HCV positive user.

The prevalence of HCV among IDU far exceeds HIV. In many countries, rates of HCV infection range between 40% and 90% (Rosen *et al.*, 2008). HCV is largely transmitted through blood to blood contact. Like HIV, the route of transmission is via shared injecting equipment, and the same factors that predict increased risk for HIV also predict risk for HCV. It is, however, a more robust virus than HIV, and more readily transmitted. The risk of contracting HCV from an episode of sharing is thus far higher than for HIV, which is why infection often occurs early in the use career (Budd *et al.*, 2002; Hagan *et al.*, 2007). Given these factors, it is not surprising that the base rate of HCV infection among IDU is substantially higher than the base rate of HIV. Unlike HIV and HBV, however, HCV is not thought to be transmitted by sexual contact.

We should not lose sight of the fact that injecting is a behaviour that carries risks for infection that extend beyond HIV and the hepatitises. Other infections may also have devastating consequences. The most prominent of these is endocarditis, an inflammation of the lining of the heart chambers and endocardium (Karch, 2009). Like the viruses discussed above, IDU contract endocarditis through the sharing of infected injecting equipment. Bacterial infection is the most common source of endocarditis, but it can also be caused by fungi. Infection may result in congestive heart failure, arrhythmias, heart valve damage, blood clots, cerebral infarction, intracranial haemorrhage and brain abscesses (Karch, 2009). HIV infection, and a previous history of endocarditis, have been found to be independent predictors of endocarditis among IDU (Karch, 2009; Spijkerman *et al.*, 1995; Zaccarelli *et al.*, 1994).

Injecting-related drug problems are not restricted to disease transmission. As discussed earlier, the injection of tablet preparations, particularly benzodiazepines and opioids such as oxycodone, has been widely documented. One sequelae of this practice is the deposition of foreign body materials within the pulmonary vasculature. This is of clinical importance, as it is associated with the development of long-term pulmonary vascular pathology, particularly pulmonary hypertension (Karch, 2009).

We know that many heroin users do not inject, although many will do so at some point. It should not be assumed, however, that avoiding injecting through heroin inhalation ('chasing') is without health risks. While associated with reduced risk of overdose and blood-borne viral infection, the practice has been associated with reduced pulmonary functioning, dyspnoea and status asthmaticus (Buster *et al.*, 2002; Cygan *et al.*, 2000). There are also documented cases of inhalation-induced leukoencephalopathy, a demylenation of the white matter of the brain, that may result in cognitive decay, seizures and death (Kriegstein *et al.*, 1999). Non-injecting users are also at risk for opioid dependence. Indeed, 10% of heroin users entering treatment in ATOS exclusively smoked heroin, and had levels of dependence equivalent to those of injectors (Darke *et al.*, 2004a).

The polydrug using nature of heroin users may expose them to risk of cardiovascular disease though the use of psychostimulants. Although psychostimulants may induce cardiovascular complications in users with normal coronary arteries, as we noted earlier, there are also long-term sequelae (Darke *et al.*, 2008a; Kaye *et al.*, 2007). In particular, the premature and accelerated development of coronary artery atherosclerosis, which increases the risk of myocardial infarction, has been associated with the chronic use of both cocaine and methamphetamine. Chronic use is also associated with ventricular hypertrophy, a condition that can predispose to methamphetamine-induced myocardial ischaemia and/or arrhythmia. As noted above, the use of psychostimulants in conjunction with opioids may increase overdose risk, particularly in the presence of severe cardiovascular pathology.

One other aspect of health and polydrug use should also be noted in passing. As we noted in Chapter 3, tobacco smoking is close to universal amongst heroin users (McCool & Richter, 2003; Ross *et al.*, 2005). In addition to all that has been discussed to date, our heroin users are also exposed to the pulmonary and cardiovascular risks associated with cigarette consumption (Karch, 2009). Certainly, this may contribute to the poor physical health of users. It may also have more specific implications for what has been discussed above. For instance, reduced pulmonary function from long-term tobacco use may compromise breathing in the presence of significant respiratory depression due to the effects of heroin. Similarly, elevated blood pressure resulting from nicotine use may increase the risk of cardiovascular accidents from psychostimulant use.

We must also bear in mind that the diet of the entrenched opioid user is typically poor (Herbert *et al.*, 1990; Noble & McCombie, 1997; Zador *et al.*, 1996). This, to some degree, reflects the financial priorities of the user. Drugs are the main priority, well ahead of food. The chaotic life of the user, including insecure accommodation and possible homelessness, also render a regular, healthy dietary intake unlikely. This has implications for all users, but has specific effects upon women, with dysmenorrhoea and amenorrhoea commonly reported by heroin using women (Schmittner *et al.*, 2005). The babies of heroin using women have lower birth weights, are slower to meet developmental milestones and have higher mortality rates than other babies (Burns *et al.*, 2010; Fajemirokun-Odudeyi *et al.*, 2006; Kakko *et al.*, 2008). If the woman was actively using opioids during her pregnancy, it is likely that the baby will be born with physiological opioid dependence, and may require detoxification (Fajemirokun-Odudeyi *et al.*, 2006; Kakko *et al.*, 2008).

Also associated with poor diet, the oral health of users is also extremely poor (Laslett *et al.*, 2008; Reece, 2007). Indeed, anecdotally this is one of the major health complaints reported by heroin users. While diet certainly contributes to poor oral health, opioids retard the saliva production that protects against dental decay and periodontitis (Abdollahi & Radfarl, 2003). The mature heroin user is also unlikely to attend a dentist, or to maintain high standards of basic personal dental care (Laslett *et al.*, 2008)

5.4.3 Psychopathology

We have seen the high rates of childhood abuse and psychopathology that precede the use of heroin. Given this, as well as poor health, regular overdoses and the stresses of the lifestyle, it is not surprising that rates of psychiatric distress amongst adult users are extremely high. Studies consistently show more than half of heroin users qualify for at least one psychiatric diagnosis other than drug dependence (Brienza *et al.*, 2000; Cacciola *et al.*, 2001; Kidorf *et al.*, 2004; Maloney *et al.*, 2010; Teesson *et al.*, 2005).

Clearly, heroin users carry a heavy burden of psychological disease, including serious mood and anxiety disorders. Lifetime rates of major depression and dysthymia are in the order of a third to half, and current rates range between a quarter to a third (Brienza *et al.*, 2000; Maloney *et al.*, 2010; Teesson *et al.*, 2005). Major depression is a seriously disabling disorder (APA, 2000). In addition to the distress to the sufferer, it has serious clinical implications for those treating opioid dependence. A third to a half of users will qualify for lifetime diagnoses of anxiety disorders (Darke & Ross, 1997; Kidorf *et al.*, 2004; Lofwall *et al.*, 2005; Mills *et al.*, 2005). In particular, extremely high levels of social phobia and PTSD are reported, as well as excess rates of generalised anxiety disorder.

The other class of disorders we see in abundance amongst heroin users are the personality disorders. These are long-term maladaptive traits, commencing in childhood (APA, 2000). The most commonly diagnosed personality disorders are ASPD, its childhood antecedent CD and borderline personality disorder (BPD). ASPD is seen in at least a third of heroin users and, indeed, in up to three-quarters in some cohorts, compared with only 4% among the general population (APA, 2000; Brooner *et al.*, 1993; Darke *et al.*, 2004c; Rouser *et al.*, 1994). The diagnosis, however, is based upon antisocial *behaviours*, such as performing illegal acts, an inability to sustain consistent work behaviour and frequent lying (APA, 2000). With heroin users, there is considerable difficulty in distinguishing between the presence of a personality disorder and behaviours generated by illegal drugs. Indeed, it has been argued that ASPD is merely a redescription of criminality, and that it is not surprising that people who commit crimes to support drug use receive the diagnosis (Darke *et al.*, 2004c; Gerstley *et al.*, 1990). In this author's opinion, the diagnosis is without clear clinical meaning for this population (and possibly for any population).

Finally, while the prevalence of BPD in the general population is approximately 2%, rates amongst heroin users range from 11% to 65% (APA, 2000; Darke *et al.*, 2004c; Trull *et al.*, 2000). This diagnosis is characterised by marked impulsivity, chronic feelings of emptiness, identity disturbance, lack of anger control, intense and frequent mood changes and life-threatening behaviours. There is thus more of a focus on psychological factors, than on ASPD. As such, there is considerably less scope for diagnostic confusion resulting from behaviours driven by drug use, rather than by personality disorder.

It is evident that our mature heroin user lives under a great pressure of psychiatric disability. This has real implications for quality of life and survival. *All* of the diagnoses discussed above are strongly related to an increased likelihood of suicide and self-harm (Harris & Barraclough, 1997). Death due to suicide, and its attendant risk factors, will be discussed in Chapter 8. There are, however, estimated to be 10–20 suicide attempts for every completed suicide (Diekstra & Gulbinat, 1993). Like heroin overdose, near misses appear to comprise the majority of incidents. Given the extent of pathology we would, sadly, expect high rates of suicide attempts. Such is indeed the case. From a wide range of countries rates of lifetime and recent suicide attempts among heroin users are in the order of 20% to 40%, and 6% to 10%, respectively (Darke *et al.*, 2004b, 2007f; Darke & Ross, 2001; Rossow & Lauritzen, 1999; Roy, 2002, 2010; Tremau *et al.*, 2008). By comparison, the population lifetime prevalence of attempted suicide is in the range of 3%–5%, with the 12-month prevalence estimated at 0.4%–2.2% (Borges *et al.*, 2000; Johnstone *et al.*, 2009). Amongst both the general population and heroin users, females are three times more likely to attempt suicide than males. It needs to be borne in mind that a previous suicide attempt is a strong predictor of subsequent attempts (Darke *et al.*, 2007f; Gibbs *et al.*, 2005; Harris & Barrclough, 1997).

The related, but distinct, behaviours comprising self-harm (the deliberate destruction of body tissue without conscious suicidal intent) are also common (Maloney *et al.*, 2010). These acts commonly include cutting and burning the skin, banging the head, picking at wounds, needle-sticking, inserting objects under the skin and self-biting. As with suicide, lifetime rates are many orders of magnitudes of those in the general population (10% to 46% vs. 2% to 4%, respectively) (Cumming *et al.*, 2006; Darke *et al.*, 2010d; Evren & Evren, 2005; Harned *et al.*, 2006; Maloney *et al.*, 2010).

The picture presented here is one of serious distress, with potentially lethal consequences. Is this inescapable? Fortunately, the answer is no. As we shall see, levels of distressing pathology decline significantly during treatment, concomitant with reductions in drug use. Indeed, even ASPD appears to get 'better', a most curious occurrence in what is characterised as a stable, lifetime disorder.

5.4.4   Social disadvantage

Given the general picture of dysfunction we have presented, it will come as no surprise that the social profile of users is also poor. Financial problems are very much the norm, and will typically emerge early in the use career (Azim *et al.*, 2008; Galea *et al.*, 2003; Neale & Robertson, 2005; Ross *et al.*, 2005). There are two reasons for this. Firstly, the daily use of illicit, and licit, drugs is extremely expensive. We would expect the typical user to be using several thousand dollars of drugs each week. Financial hardship would be difficult to avoid. It is unlikely, however, that our heroin user will be employed. Studies of street heroin users, those entering treatment and those in treatment are universal in reporting that most entrenched heroin users are unemployed, or on some form of government benefit, with rates ranging from two-thirds to over 90% (Bell *et al.*, 2009; Haasen *et al.*, 2007; Hser *et al.*, 1999; Maloney *et al.*, 2009; Ross *et al.*, 2005). Moreover, this is not merely transient unemployment. We are not simply unlucky in catching the population 'between jobs'. This is long-term, entrenched unemployment.

There are a number of reasons why the mature heroin user is likely to be unemployed. Firstly, the drug use patterns described above will severely impact upon the ability to obtain, and hold, a job. Using heroin and other substances several times a day means that the person will be affected by drugs for large proportions of the day, and is unlikely to be fit to work. Heroin is, after all, a soporific, and the use of machinery and vehicles whilst intoxicated is extremely dangerous. Secondly, as we will see below, almost all users who have been using for any length of time will have a criminal record, which will entirely preclude them from many jobs, and make it far more difficult to obtain employment in others. Related to this, the financial burden of drug use means that crime takes up a large part of the week. In an odd sense, many mature users are simply too busy committing crime, obtaining drugs, using them and recovering to be able to work.

Another factor operating against the financial stability of our heroin user is their relatively low level of educational achievement. The majority of heroin users have not completed high school, and university qualifications are rare (Coffin *et al.*, 2007; Darke *et al.*, 2010e; Flynn *et al.*, 2003; Manfredi *et al.*, 2006; Rosen *et al.*, 2008).

Finally, relevant to social disadvantage, there is a lack of housing stability among many mature users (Azim *et al.*, 2008; Coffin *et al.*, 2007; Vlahov *et al.*, 2008). Given the substantial levels of financial difficulties, and the need to spend on drugs, these levels perhaps should not surprise. The issue is, however, a vitally important one. Housing instability is known to be associated with higher levels of psychopathology and poorer health and is a risk factor for overdose and assault (Kerr *et al.*, 2007; Ochoa *et al.*, 2001).

5.4.5 Crime

The stereotypic image of the entrenched, mature heroin user is one of a regular criminal, and possibly a violent one at that. Is this a fair description? Yes and no. Yes, in the sense that heroin users *do* have extremely high levels of criminality. No, in the sense that they are not 'wedded' to crime, or that drug use is merely a manifestation of a pre-existing criminal nature.

The key model in this field is that of Goldstein (1985), who argued that the primary motivating force behind drug-related crime was economic compulsion. Thus, in terms of our heroin user, it is not heroin use *per se* which engenders heroin-related crime, but the economic burdens imposed by addiction to an expensive, illegal product. In the absence of legitimate means of financing drug use, drug users are likely to engage in acquisitive crimes, such as property crime or fraud. In terms of drug-related violence, Goldstein proposed three links: (i) the direct psychopharmacological effects of a substance, (ii) economic compulsive violence that arises from attempts to obtain money for drugs (such as robbery), and (iii) systemic violence that results from the dynamics of drug markets (e.g. violence between dealers).

It is beyond dispute that the regular heroin user is likely to be deeply involved in criminal activities. Typically, between half and three-quarters of regular heroin users have current, and regular, involvement in crime (Flynn *et al.*, 2003; Gossop *et al.*, 2000; Haasen *et al.*, 2007; Maher *et al.*, 2002; Torok *et al.*, in press). Importantly, while heroin use is illegal, these rates do not include drug use. Such levels of involvement should not surprise. As noted above, our user is now using opioids daily and is typically unemployed. The money has to come from somewhere. Indeed, in one study that specifically explored this issue, legitimate sources accounted for only 11% of income, the remainder coming from crime and prostitution (Maher *et al.*, 2002). Similarly, Ross *et al.* (2005) reported that crime was the *main* source of income for a quarter of treatment entrants (Ross *et al.*, 2005).

Such crime rates come at a heavy cost to victims and the community. They also, however, take a heavy toll on users. The conviction and prison records of heroin users testify to their involvement in crime. Almost all users who have been using for any length of time will have a conviction record (typically >90%), and at least half will have been incarcerated (Bargagli *et al.*, 2006; Cacciola *et al.*, 2001; Lofwall *et al.*, 2005; Ross *et al.*, 2005; Torok *et al.*, in press). Men are more likely to have a prison record, which may reflect the more salient role of prostitution as an income source amongst women users.

Consistent with the Goldstein viewpoint on economic imperative, acquisitive property crime is by far the most commonly committed act (Fisher *et al.*, 2004; Maher *et al.*, 2002; Manzoni *et al.*, 2006; Neale *et al.*, 2005; Ross *et al.*, 2005; Van der Zanden, 2007). This typically comprises shoplifting and robbery, with drug dealing coming in second, followed by fraud. In most cases of dealing we are talking about user–dealers (dealing conducted to support personal use) rather than high-level distribution.

Not surprisingly, when asked why they commit crime, the overwhelming response is to support drug use (Van der Zanden, 2007). The entrenched heroin user is not typically committing crime, or performing sex work, because they like to, or are innately 'criminal' or immoral. Consistent with the economic underpinning for most heroin-related crime, the strongest factor that predicts criminal behaviour is the person's level of heroin use (Flynn *et al.*, 2003; Gossop *et al.*, 2000; Lobmann & Verthein, 2009; Manzoni *et al.*, 2006; Patterson *et al.*, 2000). As the frequency of use increases, so does crime. Similarly, as use declines, crime does also. Heroin users are not wedded to crime. They do it for a single purpose: to purchase heroin. The idea that our heroin user is a career criminal is true only in so far the career co-occurs with their use career.

We should not come away with the impression that violence plays no part in these lives. Unfortunately, it is all too common. In terms of Goldstein's model, there is no direct psychopharmacological reason to suppose heroin-related violence. Unlike the psychostimulants, regular heroin use is not associated with paranoid symptomatology or violence after administration. Violence arising from crime generally arises from attempts to obtain money for drugs, and the systemic violence of drug market distribution (Darke *et al.*, 2010e; Neale *et al.*, 2005). Indeed, violent crime comes a distant fourth in frequency after property crime, dealing and fraud. This does not mean violent offending is uncommon. Neale *et al.* (2005) reported that one in five heroin users had committed a violent act in the preceding 3 months, while Darke *et al.* (2010e) found that a third of heroin users had done so in the preceding year. Importantly, the latter study showed this rate to be substantially lower than that of regular methamphetamine users, for whom there is a direct pharmacologic relationship between drug and violence. Consistent with Goldstein's 'systemic' violence, in both these studies drug dealing was a significant predictor of violent offending. It needs to be borne in mind that those who assault people also have a substantially increased risk of assault themselves, and that this is the case for heroin users as much as for anyone (Darke *et al.*, 2010e; Hodgins *et al.*, 2008; Neale *et al.*, 2005). As we shall see in Chapter 8, the criminal involvement of heroin users may have lethal consequences.

Given the high rates of criminality and ASPD, can our heroin user be characterised as a psychopath? I do not believe so. As discussed above, ASPD is a diagnosis based upon antisocial behaviours, and does not adequately distinguish between those who may be termed 'true psychopaths' and 'symptomatic psychopaths' (those who perform the behaviours as a result of substance dependence) (Gerstley *et al.*, 1990). In the only study to directly compare diagnoses of ASPD and psychopathy, half met ASPD criteria, but only 5% could be termed true 'psychopaths' (Darke *et al.*, 1998). Most heroin users perform crime because they have to, not because they want to. The strong relationship between use and crime levels makes this abundantly clear. If crime is an inherent part of the make-up of the heroin user, it is strange that it wanes and waxes in tandem with drug use. This is not to say that crime may not precede drug use. In many cases it, and those who commit crime prior to heroin use, are more likely to commit violent crime (Hall *et al.*, 1993; Kaye *et al.*, 1998). The predominant pattern, however, is of a user who has become entrenched in a cycle of drugs, crime and incarceration. Committing these crimes, however, does not make the user a psychopath.

5.5 Summary

The heroin user is now firmly entrenched in a polydrug using lifestyle, of which heroin is merely one component. The serious problems that accompany heroin dependence are emerging. As these problems worsen, the possibility of drug treatment comes into the focus of the user. In the next chapter we will discuss the cycle of treatment and relapse that characterises the career trajectories of so many heroin users.

Key points: Summary of the 20s and 30s: heroin and polydrug use

- By their 20s, the heroin user will typically be dependent and using heroin several times a day.
- Heroin use sits amidst extensive polydrug use, with the use of alcohol, benzodiazepines and the psychostimulants being of the greatest clinical interest.
- Overdose is a major problem for established heroin users, and the risk is strongly exacerbated by polydrug use.
- Mature heroin users display extremely high rates of psychopathology, including mood, anxiety, and personality disorders, and have extensive histories of attempted suicide.
- The physical health of established users is also poor, with high rates of blood-borne viral infections, poor nutrition and poor dental health.
- The established user experiences very high levels of financial and social deprivation, and most are long-term unemployed.
- Established users are very likely to engage in crime and/or sex work to support their use. The frequency of crime is directly related to the frequency of heroin use.

6

The drug treatment cycle: remission and relapse

6.1 Introduction

In the preceding chapter we saw the extensive drug use and burden of disease of the mature heroin user. The mature user is on a daily (or near daily) cycle of crime or sex work to support drug use. The demands of the lifestyle upon the user, and those around them, are difficult to maintain. Treatment offers some hope for amelioration of this chaotic lifestyle.

We will now examine treatment options for our user, the treatment cycle and the positive effects derived from treatment. While the general picture presented to date is bleak, there is certainly hope. Indeed, one of the major findings of the international literature of the past 50 years is that 'treatment works'. It is associated with substantial reductions in heroin and other drug use, as well as in reductions in the severity of a constellation of drug-related problems. Relapse rates are high, and the achievement of stable abstinence difficult, but treatment does make great improvements to the general quality of life of the dependent heroin user.

6.2 What are the main treatments for heroin dependence?

Drug treatment covers a range of different modalities and philosophies. Broadly speaking, treatment falls into three domains: detoxification, inpatient residential rehabilitation and outpatient pharmacotherapies. Traditionally, there has been a great deal of conflict between the proponents of different modalities, much of which revolves around drug-free versus medicated recovery. We in the field have been treated to this unedifying debate for decades. Heroin users, however, show far more sense, and far less ideology. They switch freely between treatment modalities, depending on motivation, need and availability (Cox & Corniskey 2007; Ross *et al.*, 2005).

Table 6.1. Signs and symptoms of the opioid withdrawal syndrome

---

- Sweating, watery eyes, rhinorhea, increased urinary frequency, diarrhoea, nausea, vomiting, abdominal cramps
- Muscle spasm resulting in headaches, backaches, leg cramps
- Piloerection (goosebumps), dilated pupils
- Elevated blood pressure, tachycardia
- Anxiety, irritability, dysphoria, sleep disturbance
- Craving for opioids

6.2.1 Detoxification

Detoxification is a short-term intervention to remove 'toxins' from the body, in this case heroin (Lintzeros *et al.*, 2009; Meader, 2010). It has been suggested that a better term to describe this process is 'withdrawal management' (Lintzeros *et al.*, 2009). The term is so entrenched, however, that it is difficult to see it dropping out of vogue. The cessation of regular heroin use is associated with an acute withdrawal syndrome, comprising physical and psychological manifestations (Table 6.1). Overall, the syndrome is phenomenologically similar to a bad cold or mild influenza. It is uncomfortable, but it is *not* life-threatening. Symptoms commence 8–12 hours after the cessation of heroin use, and typically peak on the third day following cessation (Lintzeros *et al.*, 2009). The syndrome usually resolves after a week.

The primary aim of detoxification is to interrupt the pattern of regular, heavy heroin use described previously. Managed withdrawal may occur in inpatient or outpatient environments. Subsidiary aims are to alleviate the withdrawal syndrome described above and, hopefully, link the user with other treatment or support services. Managing the amelioration of the withdrawal syndrome may be achieved through reducing doses of an opioid agonist (usually methadone), reducing doses of a partial opioid agonist (buprenorphine) and/or symptomatic relief through α_2 adrenergic agonists such as clonidine and lofexidine. To date, it would appear that the best results are obtained through the use of methadone or buprenorphine, which appear superior to the use of the α_2 adrenergic agonists alone (Meader, 2010). Moreover, buprenorphine would appear to be associated with a less severe and prolonged withdrawal, and higher rates of detoxification completion (Meader, 2010; Reed *et al.*, 2007).

Interestingly, most studies do not find a significant association between the amount of heroin being used prior to detoxification and the severity of the withdrawal syndrome (Gossop *et al.*, 1987; Phillips *et al.*, 1986;

Smolka & Schmidt, 1999). This is a probable reflection of the fact that to be motivated, or required, to enter detoxification the user would have to be dependent. What *does* consistently predict withdrawal severity, however, are patient psychological factors (Kanof *et al.*, 1993; Lintzeros *et al.*, 2009; Phillips *et al.*, 1986; Ziedonis *et al.*, 2009). A more depressed, anxious patient with expectations of a severe syndrome will, on the whole, experience more severe symptoms. It is an excellent example of a self-fulfilling prophecy.

It is doubtful that detoxification should be considered a treatment *per se* but, rather, as a route to long-term intervention. As we shall see below, it is long-term interventions that engender change. The risk of relapse to use after a successful, or unsuccessful, detoxification is high (Strang *et al.*, 2003; Teesson *et al.*, 2006a; Wines *et al.*, 2007). Unlike maintenance therapies and residential rehabilitation, there is no evidence of long-term improvement deriving from detoxification *per se*. Moreover, given the reduction in opioid tolerance, the risk of overdose in the period immediately following detoxification is elevated (Strang *et al.*, 2003; Teesson *et al.*, 2006a; Wines *et al.*, 2007). By the time they seek treatment, heroin users have typically been using heroin for a long time, and are likely to have severe problems associated with dependent use. It should not be expected that a brief, 1-week intervention will suddenly change the user's life. This would be placing naive, and unrealistic, expectations on what detoxification can achieve.

6.2.2 Drug-free residential rehabilitation

Drug-free residential rehabilitation is a major, long-term modality for the treatment of substance dependence. Unlike the substitution treatments discussed below, residential rehabilitation is *not* a treatment specifically for heroin dependence or, indeed, for dependence on any particular substance. The most well-known form of residential rehabilitation is the therapeutic community. The pioneer, and template, in the development of this treatment modality was the Synanon community, commencing in the USA in the late 1950s (Hubbard *et al.*, 1989).

As the name suggests, residential programmes involve users living in a treatment community. This is a major distinguishing feature of the modality when compared with outpatient treatment modalities, such as methadone maintenance. Entrants undergo detoxification prior to commencing residential rehabilitation. Treatment is drug free, as the name suggests, the second major distinguishing feature of the modality. Users are not medicated, as is the case in the maintenance modalities. Fundamental change in behaviour and personality is to be achieved without the use of drugs. Under the residential model, it is seen as necessary for the drug users to change their lifestyle completely. This involves abstinence from drugs, eliminating antisocial behaviours, as well as the development of employment skills, self-reliance and personal honesty. Under this paradigm, this is best achieved by a temporary withdrawal from the outside world, to a supportive treatment community. Programmes vary, but are usually from 3–12 months. Rather than focus on a specific substance, dependence (or 'addiction') *per se* is seen as the problem. Addiction is seen as a disease, whether this be for alcohol, heroin or any substance. The approach taken can thus be seen as holistic. A residential programme aims to elicit change in all aspects of the person's life, as well as all aspects of drug use, in order to produce a healthy and productive individual. In broad terms, in a therapeutic community, it is the community itself that is the therapy. Most programmes are based upon the Twelve Steps, originally developed by Alcoholics Anonymous, and broadened to cover all substances. These involve a recognition of the role of addiction in the person's life, admission of character faults and fundamental changes to the person themselves.

Residential rehabilitation treatment is always highly structured. It should be noted that the profile of entrants is of a slightly more dysfunctional group than that seen in maintenance (DeLeon *et al.*, 2008; Ross *et al.*, 2005). Indeed, it may be just this group that will benefit from a highly structured environment. Days are kept full with group sessions, individual psycho-therapy and doing work around the community (e.g. meal preparation). Participation in Narcotics Anonymous or Alcoholics Anonymous groups is often a component of treatment, and such participation is seen as a valuable support for a drug-free lifestyle after re-entry into the wider community. Treatment is staged, such that after successfully completing each stage, the individual advances to a stage that carries further responsibilities within the community, and acts as a role model for their peers. There is a strong emphasis on the development of skills for life outside the community, particularly on educational and employment skills.

As with the other long-term treatment modality, opioid maintenance, residen-tial rehabilitation has been demonstrated to be an effective form of treatment, with longer retention associated with better outcomes (Darke *et al.*, 2006b; Gossop *et al.*, 1999). Consistent with the holistic approach of such programmes, residential rehabilitation has been shown to have a broader effect upon polydrug use amongst primary heroin users than opioid maintenance treatment (Darke *et al.*, 2006b). In addition to retention *per se*, successful completion of a programme is associated with a superior outcome (Darke *et al.*, 2006b).

As with all forms of treatment, there are negatives to consider. Firstly, there is the problem of attracting users to a drug-free alternative, something the maintenance therapies do not have to deal with. This is, in all probability, why maintenance treatment has always attracted larger numbers than residential treatment. Secondly, early drop-out is a problem, as many users find it difficult to make the transition to a drug-free intervention, although this is a problem for all modalities (Gossop *et al.*, 1999; Mulder *et al.*, 2009; Ross *et al.*, 2006). Finally, relapse after treatment poses a particular problem. As we noted earlier, tolerance declines rapidly during periods of abstinence, and relapse presents a period of greatly elevated overdose risk.

6.2.3   Opioid maintenance therapies

We now turn to pharmacological maintenance. This category of treatment comprises outpatient opioid substitution, and has traditionally been the most popular of the treatment alternatives. The modality owes its existence to the pioneering work of Dole and Nyswander with methadone in the United States in the 1960s (Dole & Nyswander, 1965; Dole *et al.*, 1966). Methadone hydrochloride is a long-acting opioid agonist with a half-life of 24 hours, and is typically delivered as an oral liquid suspension (Mattick *et al.*, 2009). Tablet forms of the drug exist, but are usually administered to chronic pain patients.

The drug shows cross-tolerance with other opioids, such as heroin, and competes for the same mu opioid receptors. This means that the individual will not experience withdrawal after ceasing, or reducing, their heroin use. Essentially, methadone replaces heroin. If heroin is taken, larger amounts are needed to gain any effects, due to the presence of methadone on the mu receptors. Indeed, large methadone doses have been referred to as 'blockade', in that they effectively block the effects of other opioids. The popularity of the modality is based upon the fact that the user does not have to experience withdrawal, or go 'cold turkey', but can continue to receive an opioid. The therapeutic aim is to achieve a dose that precludes withdrawal, on which the patient is comfortable, without inducing intoxication or sedative effects (Mattick *et al.*, 2009).

The original rationale behind methadone treatment was based upon the model of insulin in the treatment of diabetes. The user was conceived as having a metabolic imbalance, requiring continuing administration of opioids. By providing a licit opioid, craving is ameliorated, and the user no longer has to use expensive, illicit drugs like heroin. As methadone treatment developed over the years, however, the role of ancillary services has been recognised, including psychosocial supports. Methadone today is not typically seen as an insulin analogue, but as a drug administered within the context of broader treatment services. In other words, treatment now more broadly reflects the dependence syndrome, rather than being focussed solely on its physiological component.

A major advantage of methadone as a treatment intervention is that its long half-life permits single daily dosing (Mattick *et al.*, 2009; Ward *et al.*, 1998). Heroin, as we have seen, has a far shorter half-life, and the dependent user typically uses the drug several times a day. By contrast, the user may go to the clinic for dosing once a day, or use take-home doses once daily. The second major therapeutic advantage of methadone is the change from injecting to oral administration. As we have seen, injecting is the most common route of administration for the long-term heroin user. A change to an oral route of administration reduces the regular vascular damage being done by the injector, and substantially reduces the risk of overdose and needle-borne infections. Even if the user is a heroin smoker, there are advantages, in that no damage is being done to the pulmonary system, and there is no risk of inhalation-induced leukoencephalopathy. Of course, there are a large number of advantages that arise simply by engaging a user in the broader health system.

One of the most important controversies across the years has concerned appropriate maintenance dosage. While originally conceived of as a blockade drug, given in daily doses exceeding 100 mg, doses vary widely across clinics and cultures. Probably the single most important finding in the literature is that higher doses are associated with longer treatment retention and better outcomes (Kritz *et al.*, 2009; Mattick *et al.*, 2009; Ward *et al.*, 1998). A therapeutic maintenance dose would appear to be at least 60 mg administered daily. Below this dose, efficacy is doubtful.

While methadone has been the maintenance drug of choice for some decades, a range of new drugs have been developed. The most important, and widely used, of these is buprenorphine. Buprenorphine is a partial opioid agonist, with antagonist properties, which has become increasingly popular as a maintenance drug for the treatment of heroin dependence (Mattick *et al.*, 2009). Indeed, in countries such as France it is by far the largest treatment modality. Due to its partial antagonist properties, and the fact that it demonstrates a ceiling effect on respiratory suppression, buprenorphine is seen as safer than methadone. The drug is dispensed in 0.4, 2.0 and 8.0 mg sublingual tablets, and is also available in a combined preparation of buprenorphine and naloxone (the opioid antagonist used to reverse opioid overdose)

(Bell *et al.*, 2004, 2007). The naloxone is inactive, unless the preparation is injected by the user, in which case they will undergo acute opioid withdrawal. Like methadone, buprenorphine is a long-acting opioid. The major advantage of buprenorphine is that alternate day dosing may be employed, leaving the user not as tied to the clinic as is the case with daily dosing (Mattick *et al.*, 2009). Buprenorphine has been shown to be as efficacious as methadone as a maintenance drug, so it offers a real alternative (Lintzeros *et al.*, 2004; Mattick *et al.*, 2003, 2009). The withdrawal syndrome is also not as severe as that associated with methadone. As with methadone, better retention and outcomes are associated with higher maintenance doses (Ahmadi *et al.*, 2004; Ling *et al.*, 1998; Mattick *et al.*, 2009).

It should also be noted in passing that heroin itself has also been trialled as a maintenance drug (Bammer, 2009; Perneger *et al.*, 1998; Rehm *et al.*, 2001; van den Brink *et al.*, 2003). The rationale is similar to other maintenance treatments in providing an alternative opioid to use in a safe environment, except that in this case the treatment is providing 'clean' heroin to users. It also aims to attract those who would not otherwise consider treatment, or could be classified as treatment failures. Trials report users being successfully recruited (particularly long-term 'hard cases'), and reduction in drug use and crime (Bammer, 2009; Perneger *et al.*, 1998; Rehm *et al.*, 2001; van den Brink *et al.*, 2003). It is difficult, however, to see heroin maintenance becoming a major form of treatment for heroin dependence. The major reason for this is a societal and political aversion to giving heroin to heroin users. The provision of injectable grade heroin is also far more expensive than the provision of oral methadone or buprenorphine.

There are also clinical issues to consider regarding the use of heroin itself as a maintenance drug. The major advantage of drugs such as methadone and buprenorphine is that they have longer half-lives than heroin, so once daily or even alternate day dosing is possible. Heroin, in contrast, would usually be administered on several occasions per day. Secondly, heroin maintenance is often, but not always, by injection (Bammer, 2009). The highly dysfunctional group to whom heroin maintenance has been directed are very likely to be injectors. As discussed above, a major advantage of both methadone and buprenorphine is the transition *away* from injecting. It is possible that heroin maintenance may prove to be a useful entry to other forms of treatment. In and of itself, however, it is likely to remain a minority treatment.

The major controversy surrounding all maintenance treatments is philosophical. Many people are uncomfortable with treating heroin addiction by administering an opioid. It is claimed that this is not treating the underlying addiction. Indeed, some see it as simple social control and the term 'liquid handcuffs' is sometimes used disparagingly. Several points need to be made. Firstly, the efficacy of substitution maintenance treatments for heroin dependence is unassailable. Given the fact that drugs are being administered, and controversial ones at that, the modality has been extensively studied. This treatment modality works. Heroin use and death rates substantially reduce. While many *will* continue to use heroin while on methadone or buprenorphine, they will do so at reduced rates and risk. Secondly, it is the most popular modality amongst heroin users. In my opinion, there is an ethical duty to provide a popular, effective treatment to those who desire it.

This does not mean that maintenance treatments are without negatives, some of which are serious. Firstly, methadone withdrawal is a far more protracted process than heroin withdrawal, due to the longer half-life of the drug. Whereas heroin withdrawal symptoms persist for around 7 days, the methadone withdrawal syndrome is in the order of 21 days (Gossop *et al.*, 1987; Mattick *et al.*, 2009). Agonist treatment also involve the prescription of drugs that may cause death. Of course, the active heroin user is already using dangerous drugs, and the risk of death in maintenance treatment is substantially reduced. Deaths do occur, however (Darke *et al.*, 2010a). It must be borne in mind that methadone, even in therapeutic doses, suppresses respiratory rates and oxygenation (Lintzeros *et al.*, 2006, 2007; White & Irvine, 1999). In one recent Australian study, one in six opioid toxicity deaths were methadone-related (Darke *et al.*, 2010a). Moreover, there is diversion of maintenance drugs to the non-treatment population, so a large proportion of maintenance drug deaths occur amongst those not being treated (Darke *et al.*, 2010a). The injection of diverted methadone syrup is also well documented, a practice associated with substantial vascular damage and high overdose risk (Darke *et al.*, 1996a; Humeniuk *et al.*, 2003). It is important to note that deaths are not restricted to methadone. Buprenorphine toxicity deaths also occur, although the rate of such deaths is thought to be lower than that of methadone (Auriacombe *et al.*, 2001; Bell *et al.*, 2009; Gibson & Degenhardt, 2007).

The long-term aim of maintenance treatment is not always clear. Is it simply to keep dosing for ever? In some cases, this may be the most beneficial regime, as it is well demonstrated that a pre-emptory removal from treatment is associated with far higher risks of relapse and death (Anglin *et al.*, 1989). Is it to achieve abstinence from all opioids, including the maintenance drug? How does one make such a transition from daily medication to total opioid abstinence? These are crucial clinical decisions that do not appear to be consistent across clinics or countries.

6.2.4 Antagonist maintenance therapies

Maintenance treatments do not all involve agonist substitution. An alternative maintenance regime is based upon the provision of the opioid antagonist naltrexone hydrochloride. An opioid antagonist is a substance that, if taken in regular maintenance doses, suppresses the effects of opioids. Naltrexone binds to the mu receptors in the brain, attenuating or blocking the effects of opioids. Interestingly, naltrexone is used for the treatment of both opioid and alcohol dependence. The drug is available in tablet form, but in more recent years sustained release depot implants have become available (Kunøe et al., 2009).

To date, naltrexone has not been taken up in large numbers by heroin users (Gibson & Ritter, 2009). Induction rates into treatment are low and, given the choice, users overwhelmingly opt for the other modalities (Gibson *et al.*, 2003; Rothenberg *et al.*, 2002; Tucker *et al*, 2004). Heroin users need to be highly motivated to achieve abstinence to take a substance that blocks all effects of opioids. For such highly motivated individuals, however, naltrexone may clearly be of value (Kirchmayer *et al.*, 2002; Mattick *et al.*, 2009; Minozzi *et al.*, 2006). For instance, a user who has to demonstrate heroin abstinence to a court through regular urinalysis may be highly motivated to undertake, and comply with, such treatment. For the more typical heroin user, however, strong external motivations are often lacking.

The problem with poor motivation for oral antagonist treatment is manifested in high early drop-out rates and poor compliance. Early attrition is high, and retention times are lower than those seen in the agonist treatment modalities (Bartu *et al.*, 2002; Gibson & Ritter, 2009; Rothenberg *et al.*, 2002). Indeed, the average retention time on naltrexone maintenance is in the order of 3 months (Gibson & Ritter, 2009). Poor compliance with an antagonist drug has implications for overdose if relapse were to occur. As discussed earlier, opioid tolerance declines rapidly during periods of abstinence, so any relapse carries a far higher risk of overdose. There is evidence of increased rates of both fatal and non-fatal overdose among patients during, and soon after leaving, naltrexone treatment (Digiusto *et al.*, 2004; Gisbon & Degenhardt, 2007; Miotto *et al.*, 1997; Oliver *et al.*, 2005; Tucker *et al.*, 2004). The new implantable depot formulations of naltrexone may well improve compliance and reduce overdose risk. Motivating users to undertake this treatment modality is likely, however, to prove difficult. In all probability, naltrexone maintenance will remain a minority option for the management of opioid dependence, and most likely to be attractive to the highly motivated user.

6.3   The treatment cycle

We have examined the treatment options available for heroin users. We must now examine the treatment cycle. The drug-related problems that we have been discussing do not arise overnight. It will take some time for them to develop to a level of severity that will motivate treatment seeking. The average age of the first treatment enrolment for heroin dependence is in the early to mid-20s, approximately 5 or so years after the initiation of heroin use, and 3 years after the development of dependence (Anglin *et al.*, 1986; Bargagli *et al.*, 2006; Hser, 1999, 2007a; Hubbard *et al.*, 1989; Luty *et al.*, 2003; McGlothlin & Anglin 1981; Oppenheimer *et al.*, 1990; Ross *et al.*, 2005). There is some evidence that women may first seek treatment at a slightly younger age than men, although the difference is only in the order of a year or so (Bargagli *et al.*, 2006; Hubbard *et al.*, 1989; Ross *et al.*, 2005).

In terms of chronology, it is extremely unlikely that this will be the sole treatment episode, followed by a complete recovery. The majority of users in treatment cohorts have previously been treated, and usually on multiple occasions (Bargagli *et al.*, 2006; Cox & Corniskey, 2010; Gossop *et al.*, 1998; Haasen *et al.* 2007; Hser *et al.*, 1999; Hubbard *et al.*, 1997; Joe *et al.*, 1999; Ross *et al.*, 2005). The heavy previous exposure in outcome studies reflects the fact that treatment cohorts generally have mean ages in the late 20s to early 30s. It should also be noted that those with treatment histories often report enrolment across many different modalities (Cox & Corniskey 2007; Haasen *et al.*, 2007; Ross *et al.*, 2005). Users appear to move freely between treatment modalities.

6.4   What does successful treatment achieve?

6.4.1   Drug use

Enrolment in the major treatment modalities is associated with large reductions in heroin use (e.g. Darke *et al.*, 2005c, 2007d; Gossop *et al.*, 2002a; Hubbard *et al.*, 1989, 1997; Simpson & Sells, 1982; Teesson *et al.*, 2007). At 12 months, UK treatment patients reported an increase in heroin abstinence from 21% to 48% (Gossop *et al.*, 2002a), while Spanish patients reported an increase from 5% to 50% (Sanchez-Carbonell *et al.*, 1988). Similarly, in the USA weekly or more frequent heroin use has been seen to reduce from 89% to 28% by 12 months (Flynn *et al.*, 2003; Hubbard *et al.*, 1997), with similarly large reductions in heroin use having been reported in other US-based studies (cf. Hubbard *et al.*, 1989; Simpson & Sells, 1982). Amongst the

ATOS cohort, approximately two-thirds were currently heroin abstinent at each of the 3, 12, 24 and 36 month follow-ups (Darke *et al.*, 2007d; Teesson *et al.*, 2007). Moreover, treatment response tends to be rapid, with substantial reductions in heroin use typically seen in the first few months of treatment, amongst both inpatients and community-based patients (Gossop *et al.*, 2002a; Hubbard *et al.*, 1989; Ross *et al.*, 2005).

Whilst the point prevalence of heroin abstinence (usually 1 or 3 months) in treatment studies looks impressive, the *maintenance* of abstinence is far more problematic (Darke *et al.*, 2005c; Hser *et al.*, 2001; Sheehan *et al.*, 1993; Simpson & Sells, 1990). Abstinence for a 1-month period may not truly reflect heroin use patterns over the entire follow-up period, and relapse appears common. Indeed, a 1-month period of abstinence may be an *exception* in the use career, rather than a reflection of sustained abstinence. Sheehan *et al.* (1993), for instance, reported that three-quarters of heroin users who entered treatment were abstinent at 12 months follow-up, but only a quarter had been abstinent for more than 80% of the time. Amongst ATOS clients, while two-thirds were abstinent at any one point, these were not always the same people. The proportion who had sustained heroin abstinence since baseline was 14% at 12 months, and 8% by 36 months (Darke *et al.*, 2007d). In the longest follow-up of heroin users conducted to date, Hser *et al.* (2001) reported that only half had maintained abstinence for more than 5 years across 33 years of follow-up. We should not lose hope, however, as there is a tendency for longer periods of abstinence to occur with repeated treatment, and we know that many users do cease use altogether (Darke *et al.*, 2007d; Hser, 2007).

As we have seen, heroin use typically occurs within the context of widespread polydrug use, and high proportions of primary heroin users meet diagnostic criteria for dependence on other drugs. While treatment may reduce heroin use, there is no evidence that reduced heroin use is accompanied by substitutive increases in other drug use. In fact, reductions in polydrug use tend to accompany reductions in heroin use (Darke *et al.*, 2006c; DeMaria *et al.*, 2000; Goldstein & Herrara, 1995; Gossop *et al.*, 2002a; Hser *et al.*, 2007a; Hubbard *et al.*, 1997). The reductions in polydrug use are reflected in the types of medications obtained by users, with significant decreases seen in treatment in the proportions obtaining prescribed benzodiazepines and narcotic analgesics (Darke *et al.*, 2007b). Such reductions in polydrug use may not be universal, as there may be variations by drug class. Alcohol looks to be particularly intransigent, with a number of studies reporting no decline in alcohol use among treated heroin users (e.g. Darke *et al.*, 2006c; Fairbank *et al.*, 1993; Gossop *et al.*, 2002a). There may also be differences between the effects of different treatment modalities upon other drug use. Both Darke *et al.* (2006c) and Hubbard *et al.* (1997), for example, reported that residential rehabilitation had more effect upon other drug use than did outpatient methadone maintenance. These findings, in all probability, reflect the pharmacological focus of maintenance upon reductions in heroin use, whereas residential rehabilitation adopts a holistic, abstinence oriented approach.

6.4.2   Drug-related problems

It would be hoped that reducing drug use would also ameliorate the severity of many of the other substantial problems faced by heroin users. This is certainly the case, as treatment is associated with improvements in psychosocial functioning and health. One of the direct positive sequelae of reduced rates of heroin and polydrug use is a substantial reduction in overdose rates (Darke *et al.*, 2007e; Seal *et al.*, 2001; Stewart *et al.*, 2002). Indeed, fatal heroin overdose cases are rarely in treatment at the time of death (Darke *et al.*, 2000; Davidson *et al.*, 2003). A reduction in overdose morbidity and mortality is not surprising, as we have seen that heroin overdoses are associated with more frequent use (Backmund *et al.*, 2009; Darke *et al.*, 2007e; Seal *et al.*, 2001; Sergeev *et al.*, 2003; Yin *et al.*, 2007). Given the role of other drugs in what are termed heroin overdoses, the reduced use of other drugs will also contribute to lower overdose rates.

A second positive sequelae of reduced rates of drug use is that rates of injecting, and needle sharing, decline (Gossop *et al.*, 2002a; Teesson *et al.*, 2006b, 2008). As with overdose, we know that more frequent use is associated with greater risk, in this case the risk of sharing injecting equipment. Given that more frequent sharing increases the risk of contracting bloodborne viruses, one positive result of treatment is a reduced risk of infection, both for the individual and others. Even without sharing equipment, reductions in needle use are beneficial in reducing vascular harm to the individual associated with injecting *per se*, as reflected in improvements in injection-related health problems in treatment.

While the primary aim of drug treatment is to treat drug use, not to reduce crime, reductions in criminality are one of the major social benefits of treatment. It is also a major political advantage in obtaining community and government support for treatment programmes. This will also reduce the risk of violence to the client, and of arrest and incarceration. As discussed in Chapter 5, extensive acquisitive property crime is performed to support heroin use.

As use decreases during treatment, so does the rate of crime (Ball *et al.*, 1991; Flynn *et al.*, 2003; Gossop *et al.*, 2002a; Hubbard *et al.*, 1997; Lobmann & Verthein, 2009; Manzoni *et al.*, 2006; Patterson *et al.*, 2000; Teesson *et al.*, 2006b, 2007).

We know that the mature user seeking treatment is very likely to have some, or multiple, forms of psychopathology. We cannot realistically expect treatment to affect the long-term maladaptive traits that comprise the various forms of personality disorder. Indeed, it is a moot question whether these can be changed (or in some cases even exist). Levels of personal distress, however, are an entirely different matter. Studies indicate that treatment for heroin dependence significantly reduces levels of psychological distress, and of depression in particular (Dean *et al.*, 2004; Gossop *et al.*, 2002a; Havard *et al.*, 2006; Hubbard *et al.*, 1997). Clinically significant improvements may be evident within the very early stages of treatment, generally in the first 3 months (Darke *et al.*, 2009b; Dean *et al.*, 2004; Ross *et al.*, 2006; Strain *et al.*, 1991). There is also limited evidence that rates of attempted suicide also decline (Darke *et al.*, 2007f, 2009b).

We should not, however, be too starry eyed about these outcomes. Whilst significant positive impacts upon psychological distress are associated with treatment, levels of psychopathology amongst treated samples remain higher than population norms. Indeed, the annual rate of attempted suicide for the ATOS cohort, after 36 months of extensive treatment, was still *five* times higher than that of the general population (Darke *et al.*, 2007f). Psychopathology is deep seated amongst heroin users, with roots going back to childhood and adolescence. We cannot expect drug treatment to ameliorate all such pathology. Reductions in drug use and the associated increase in stability of life, however, do appear to produce large improvements in mental health.

Finally, one of the consistent findings of outcome studies is that treatment is associated with substantial improvements in health (Gossop *et al.*, 2002a; Hubbard *et al.*, 1997; Salamina *et al.*, 2010; Teesson *et al.*, 2007). Amongst the ATOS cohort, for instance, global health improved from more than half a standard deviation below the population average to the average by 24 months (Teesson *et al.*, 2007). An improvement in general health should not surprise when viewed in conjunction with the reductions in injecting, drug use, increasing life stability and improvements in mental health. Generally, greater stability may mean improvements in dietary and sleep habits. Also, one major clinical benefit of treatment enrolment is that the user will have access to regular medical treatment. Reduced rates of injecting also mean that there will be a reduced risk of exposure to infection, of particular relevance to a HIV positive, immune compromised individual. As noted earlier, there is evidence that heroin use *per se* enhances HCV viral replication (Li *et al.*, 2007). Given the high rates of HCV infection, reductions in heroin use, by any route of administration, may result in improved health for the HCV positive user.

6.5   What predicts remission and relapse?

Successful treatment has been demonstrated to provide enormous clinical improvements, at least whilst the person is enrolled. Are there factors that predict good versus poor outcomes? Not surprisingly, a great deal of research has gone into this question, and a number of factors have been identified. These fall into two broad groups: those relating to the characteristics of clients, and those relating to treatment.

6.5.1   Client characteristics

Treatment clients are not an homogenous group, and poorer treatment outcome has been associated with a range of client factors. Firstly, poorer outcomes have been associated with heavier heroin use, injecting and more extensive polydrug use (Darke *et al.*, 2005c, 2007d; Flynn *et al.*, 2003; Hser *et al.*, 1998, 1999; Hubbard *et al.*, 1997; Joe *et al.*, 1988, 1999; Sanchez-Carbonell *et al.*, 1988; Simpson *et al.*, 1997). The fact that heavier heroin use is associated with poorer outcomes is intuitively sensible, as it is a measure of problem severity. We would expect heavier entrenchment in heroin use, and injecting, to be more difficult to treat, and such is the case.

Predictive drug use patterns, however, range beyond heroin use. The extent of polydrug use in and of itself is strongly predictive of poorer clinical profiles, and can be seen as a proxy for more serious drug entrenchment and problem severity. Some substances, however, have particular salience. In particular, benzodiazepine use is associated with more frequent heroin overdoses and needle sharing, more extensive polydrug use, as well as poorer physical and psychological health (Darke *et al.*, 2010c; Ghitza *et al.*, 2008; Kerr *et al.*, 2007). Similarly, cocaine use is also strongly associated with a poorer profile, including more frequent injections, needle sharing, sexual risk-taking and a higher prevalence of HIV (Chaisson *et al.*, 1989; Doherty *et al.*, 2000; Williamson *et al.*, 2007).

The other major non-drug factor that predicts poor outcome is heavier criminal involvement (Darke *et al.*, 2005c; Flynn *et al.*, 2003; Hser *et al.*, 1999;

Joe *et al.*, 1998; Sanchez-Carbonell *et al.*, 1988). This finding, in all probability, relates to the drug use patterns just discussed. As we have seen, levels of crime are directly related to levels of substance use. We would expect the more severe profile user, who is using large amounts of heroin and other drugs, to have a heavier level of criminal involvement, if only from economic necessity. It is unlikely to be criminality *per se* that relates to a poorer outcome, but the fact that it is a proxy for a more severely dependent user.

The picture to date of a poorer prognosis is one of greater problem severity, reflected in drug use and crime. A further factor that relates to this is the finding that a history of previous treatment predicts poor outcomes (Anglin *et al.*, 1997; Darke *et al.*, 2005c, 2007d; Hser *et al.*, 1999). Why this would be the case is not immediately apparent. It might be assumed, for instance, that a first treatment is more likely to fail. The finding is a probable reflection of the more severe drug use characteristics of repeat treatment seekers, and is thus a marker for more severe drug problems.

One other factor that has received a great deal of attention is psychological distress. Psychological distress, however, has been an inconsistent predictor of treatment outcome. While some studies report an association with poorer outcomes (Darke *et al.*, 2007d; Hser, 2007; Joe *et al.*, 1998), others report no association, particularly in relation to continued drug use (Ball & Ross, 1991; Cacciola *et al.*, 2001; Cecile *et al.*, 2001; Darke *et al.*, 2005c; Mulder *et al.*, 2009). The picture remains unclear, and may reflect the different contributions of various forms of psychopathology to outcomes. It may also reflect the fact that baseline rates are so high amongst this population. Certainly, psychological distress should not automatically be seen as a marker for poor outcome.

Personality disorders, however, are a different matter. Both ASPD and BPD are associated with higher levels of risky and harmful behaviours, and poorer treatment outcome (Brooner *et al.*, 1993; Darke *et al.*, 2004c, 2005d, 2007c; Hatzitaskos *et al.*, 1999; Rutherford *et al.*, 1994; Schaar & Ojehagan, 2001). As discussed previously, however, there are serious doubts about what the diagnosis of ASPD actually signifies, as it is based upon a range of antisocial behaviours. BPD, however, is far more psychologically based. While both predict poor outcomes, ASPD and BPD are highly coextensive (Darke *et al.*, 2004c). When directly compared, however, it has been shown that it is BPD that is the diagnosis that makes the most significant contribution to risk and poor outcomes (Darke *et al.*, 2004c).

Finally, the 'treatment readiness' of clients, or motivation to change, has been posited as a major influence on treatment outcome (Broome *et al.*, 1999;

Darke *et al.*, 2005c; Flynn *et al.*, 2003; Joe *et al.*, 1998). The willingness of clients to engage in treatment, and to actively attempt to alter their drug use behaviours appears to be a crucial component behind successful treatment. It is difficult to treat someone who does not wish to change. Treatment, and the cessation of drug use, is a difficult process, and motivation is crucial to success. The model most often mentioned in relation to treatment readiness is the Transtheoretical Model, or Stages of Change (Prochaska *et al.*, 1985; Prochaska & Velicer, 1997). The classical model postulates six distinct stages of treatment readiness amongst drug users: (i) precontemplation, (ii) preparation, (iii) contemplation, (iv) action, (v) maintenance and, finally, (vi) termination of use. Individuals progress through these stages sequentially. They may, however, regress before finally advancing to maintenance and termination. While widely used as a marker for treatment readiness, it should be borne in mind that the model has been heavily criticised (West, 2005, 2006). The basic criticism is that the concept of distinct stages is arbitrary, as are the dividing lines between them. It also relies on people making conscious decisions about their lives and drug use, a highly questionable tenet. It could also well be argued that the stages are tautological, being mere redescriptions of obvious behaviours: I am not interested in treatment so I am a 'precontemplator', I am entering treatment so I am taking 'action'. The motivational dynamics of treatment readiness are still not well understood, and more satisfying theoretical models need to be developed to understand these processes. Regardless of theoretical niceties, however, the willingness of an individual to seek treatment and active changes in their lives is clearly crucial.

6.5.2   Treatment characteristics

Some of the factors that relate to individual modalities have been discussed above. Thus, higher doses in agonist maintenance treatment are associated with better outcomes, as is successful graduation in residential rehabilitation. There are, however, a few general characteristics of successful treatment that apply across modalities. The major factor that has emerged is that longer retention times are consistently associated with better outcomes (Darke *et al.*, 2005c, 2007d; Flynn *et al.*, 2003; Gossop *et al.*,1999; Hubbard *et al.*, 1997; Kritz *et al.*, 2009; Sanchez-Carbonell *et al.*, 1988; Simpson *et al.*, 1997; Teesson *et al.*, 2007). Importantly, this is not a modality specific finding, being true for both maintenance and drug-free rehabilitation. Effectively, longer retention times mean that the client receives a larger 'treatment dose', by which we mean overall exposure to the treatment regime (Joe *et al.*, 1999).

The picture is, however, more complex than a simple accumulation of time in treatment. It is *stable retention* that is the key. While *longer* retention times are associated with better outcomes, so are *fewer* treatment episodes (Darke *et al.*, 2005c, 2007d; Gossop *et al.*, 1999). An effective treatment 'dose' does not equate to cumulative time in any number of treatment episodes. Thus, the clinical profile of someone who spent a large number of treatment days over multiple enrolments will typically be poorer than the person who spent the same number of days in a single enrolment. The best results are seen amongst those who have spent long periods in a single enrolment.

It is the efficacy of long-term, stable retention that explains why detoxification, in and of itself, is not associated with positive treatment outcomes. As discussed above, detoxification is a short-term intervention, typically around a week. It has previously been reported that retention times of at least 90 days are required for positive treatment outcomes (Hubbard *et al.*, 1997). Detoxification *per se* would not appear to supply a sufficient 'treatment dose' to engender sustained abstinence. While detoxification may act as a gateway to other treatment, by itself there is no evidence that it acts as a sustained clinical intervention. This should not surprise. The clinical profile of the mature heroin user is severe, and many of these problems have their roots deep in childhood. It is unrealistic to expect a brief detoxification to ameliorate the long-standing, severe problems we have examined. This is certainly not to say that detoxification is without merit. We should not, however, place unrealistic expectations upon the process. Simply removing a substance form the blood does not change long-standing pathology.

6.6 Summary

In the space of only some 5 or so years, the heroin user has progressed from the initiation of heroin use, the development of dependence and has enrolled in treatment. By any standards, this is a remarkably quick progression, and demonstrates the severe dependence liability of this drug. It is certainly true that most heroin users will enter treatment, and will do so on numerous occasions. The fact that a cycle of treatment and relapse occurs should not blind us to the enormous benefits that treatment confers. Even if relapses occur, time in treatment extends the life of the user, and substantially improves the quality of that life. Moreover, many will eventually achieve sustained abstinence. Events do not, however, continue at the pace that have seen to date. The chronicity of heroin dependence must always be kept in mind. In the next chapter we will examine that most forgotten of groups, the older heroin user, and the clinical issues that they face.

Key points: Summary of the drug treatment cycle: remission and relapse

- The major treatment modalities are detoxification, residential rehabilitation, opioid maintenance therapies and opioid antagonist therapies.
- The average age of first treatment enrolment is in the early to mid-20s, 5 or so years after heroin initiation.
- Multiple treatment enrolments are the norm. More than half of treatment entrants are re-enrolments.
- Users move freely between treatment modalities.
- Enrolment in treatment is associated with large reductions in heroin use. Sustained abstinence, however, occurs amongst a minority.
- Polydrug use also declines with treatment. There is no convincing evidence for drug substitution as heroin use declines.
- Treatment is associated with declines in overdose, injecting and needle sharing.
- Treatment reduces rates of criminality and psychopathology and improves health status.
- Client characteristics associated with poor outcome include heavier heroin use, injecting, more extensive polydrug use, heavier criminal involvement, previous treatment history, some forms of psychopathology and poor motivation to change.
- The most important treatment characteristic associated with positive outcomes is stable retention. Longer retention times and fewer treatment episodes are associated with better outcomes.

7

The older heroin user: the 40s and beyond

7.1 Introduction

If they have survived, our heroin user will by now have been using for something like 20 years. Many users, however, will not live to this age. Surviving is not an easy process for the long-term heroin user, as we shall see in the next chapter. By the age we are now discussing, we would expect half of those who commenced heroin use to be deceased (Hser *et al.*, 2007a). What of the survivors, however? Are there many active users by this age, or will they have typically 'matured out' after cycles of drug use, treatment, relapse and recovery? In this chapter we will examine the older heroin user. Do they exist in large numbers? After so many years of heroin use, and the significant harms associated with such use, what is the physical and psychological health of the older user like? Are there specific health and treatment issues that relate to such users? We will first examine the 'maturing out' hypothesis, the evidence relating to it and then move on to address the health and psychological profiles of the older user.

7.2 Do heroin users 'mature out'?

7.2.1 The 'maturing out' hypothesis

Maturing out may be viewed as the late career counterpart to the gateway hypothesis discussed earlier. While gateway theory examines the road *into* addiction, the maturing out hypothesis examines the path *out* of addiction. The term 'maturing out' is applied to the concept of heroin addicts outgrowing their drug habits, and was first posited by Winick in the early 1960s (Anglin *et al.*, 1986; Hser *et al.*, 2007b; Temorshuizen *et al.*, 2005; Winick, 1962). Winick's theory is that heroin users typically cease use as they get older, because the social pressures that motivated the addiction became less salient, or were more readily dealt with by the mature user. Two distinct processes were posited that produced maturation: age and length of career. Cessation of heroin use was seen as a function of the lifecycle (age) and of the course of the disease (length of drug use career) (Winick, 1964).

Like gateway theory, the origins of the theory were data driven. In examining Federal Bureau of Narcotics' records, Winick (1962) noted that those who became heroin users in their late teens ceased to appear on public health records between their mid-20s to mid-30s. The majority were alive and had ceased use, and assumed 'normal' societal roles. The average duration of addiction was reported as just under 9 years.

The maturation hypothesis certainly has great intuitive appeal. It seems to make sense that use would diminish with age, as this is what we see with so many other behaviours of the teens and 20s. As we will see below, however, there are serious limitations to this theory. In particular, as heroin use has become more entrenched in societies, the dominant trajectory of the dependent heroin user does not approximate that seen in the maturation hypothesis. Rather, long-term use into the fifth and sixth decades of life now appears common.

7.3 Drug use patterns of the older heroin user

One of the first things that should be noted about the maturing out hypothesis is that it was posited prior to the rise of heroin as a major illicit drug in western industrialised societies during the late 1960s, and prior to the baby boomer generation having reached maturity. This generation is of particular note, as substance use amongst this demographic is far in excess of that seen in previous generations, a trend that has continued in subsequent cohorts. Firstly let us briefly examine the epidemiological data. There was a pronounced ageing of populations in western industrialised societies over the course of the twentieth and early twenty-first centuries, which is still continuing (Firoz & Carlson, 2004; Gossop & Moos, 2008). This is due to longer life expectancies, and the ageing of the demographic bubble represented by the baby boomer generation, born between 1946 and 1964. For instance, in Europe the number of people aged 65 or more has trebled over the course of the twentieth century, and by 2050 a third of Europeans will be aged over 60 (Gossop & Moos, 2008).

Is an ageing population likely to translate into larger numbers of older illicit drug users, or will we simply see more 'mature' older people and, thus, less drug use? The answer appears to be the former. There have been substantial increases in the numbers of older drug users, and a steadily increasing demand for substance abuse treatment amongst older people (Beynon *et al.*, 2009; Firoz & Carlson, 2004; Gossop & Moos, 2008; Hamilton & Grella, 2009; Hartel *et al.*, 2006; Lofwall *et al.*, 2005; Rosen *et al.*, 2008).

The assumption that older people 'grow out' of drug use, the basis of the maturing out hypothesis, appears to have been based upon the misconception that older people do not use drugs (Lofwall *et al.*, 2005). This may well have been the case in days of yore, but the evidence is clear that this no longer applies. Even in that time, however, many of the users in Winick's data did not necessarily cease use, but became better at avoiding detection through the use of pharmaceutical opioids, as reported in the oral histories from Courtwright *et al.* (1990). There are now far more older people, and far more older drug users. It is projected that the number of US illicit drug users aged over 50 years old who require drug treatment will more than double between 2001 and 2020 (Beynon *et al.*, 2009; Lofwall *et al.*, 2005). Similarly, in Europe those receiving drug treatment who are aged over 65 years will double across this period (Beynon *et al.*, 2009). These trends are already evident. In the US state of Maryland, there was a 350% increase between 1988 and 2003 in methadone patients aged over 50 (Lofwall *et al.*, 2005). Again in the USA, between 1994 and 2004 the proportion of those over 50 enrolled in treatment for heroin dependence tripled (Rosen *et al.*, 2008). Indeed, by the end of that decade, the 40–50-year-old demographic was the largest cohort in treatment, constituting a quarter of those enrolled (Rosen *et al.*, 2008).

At a population level, at any rate, there appears to be ample evidence that maturation out of drug use does not occur for a great many people. The population data most certainly do *not* look like people are maturing out in their 20s and early 30s. Indeed, all the major population trends are moving in the opposite direction. If the 40–50-year-old demographic is the largest cohort in heroin treatment, their 'maturation' is rather slow in coming. We must now specifically examine our target population, the heroin user.

Support for the maturation hypothesis appears restricted to studies of heroin users conducted in the early 1960s, representing a cohort from the 1950s (Robins, 1993; Winick, 1962, 1964). Returned Vietnam veterans also demonstrated this trajectory (Robins, 1993), but this was most unusual in that they became dependent whilst in Vietnam, where heroin was plentiful and

cheap, but returned home to an entirely different situation. They had, effectively, 'done a geographical' as users put it when they move away from their
supply sources. Since then, as the heroin epidemic has progressed and use has
become embedded in western societies, the evidence for maturation is scant.
The most prominent study of long-term heroin use patterns was the 33-year
follow-up of Hser and colleagues (Hser *et al.*, 2001, 2007a). At their most
recent follow-up, the cohort were aged in their 50s. Of survivors, 20% had
opiate positive urines, and less than half had maintained heroin abstinence for
more than 5 years. Hser *et al.* (2007a) reported three distinct career trajectories: stable high-level users who constituted the majority (59%) of the cohort, a
'decelerated' group of 32% who maintained use for 10 years then tapered off,
and a much smaller group of 'early quitters' (9%) who ceased use within
7 years. Contrary to maturing out, the dominant trajectory was the long-term,
high-level user. The maturation hypothesis would predict that the overwhelming majority of the cohort should have been ex-users after so long. This was,
however, a minority trajectory. Other longitudinal studies have produced
similar evidence of long-term stable use, in contrast to the maturation model
(Goldstein & Harrara, 1995; Hamilton & Grella, 2009; Hartel *et al.*, 2006;
Rathod *et al.*, 2005; Temorshuizen *et al.*, 2005). In another 33-year follow-up,
Rathod *et al.* (2005) reported that 20% of survivors were enrolled in methadone maintenance. In their 22-year follow-up, Goldstein & Harrara (1995)
reported that 41% of survivors were still using heroin, and 48% were in
treatment. Also at 20 years, Temorshuizen *et al.* (2005) found three-quarters
of survivors were still using heroin.

Two cross-sectional studies that specifically examined older heroin users
(over 50) reported findings similar to those of the longitudinal research
(Hamilton & Grella, 2009; Hartel *et al.*, 2006). Hamilton & Grella (2009)
reported that over half of their sample had engaged in illegal drug use in the
past year. They specifically noted that chronic users do *not* mature out, but are
motivated by life events to continue their use or to cease. Similarly, Hartel
et al. (2006) found that, of surviving heroin users over 50, 40% were using
drugs, 19% were using heroin and 41% were in treatment for heroin dependence. The comments and data mirror those of Simpson and colleagues in the
early 1990s, who argued that motivations for change only appear when the
costs and problems directly associated with addiction begin to outweigh its
benefits (Simpson & Sells, 1990). It is not maturation that is relevant, but the
balance of positive and negative life events.

Consistent with the longitudinal data, age and length of career are not
predictors of cessation (Darke *et al.*, 2005c, 2006, 2007; Hser, 2007; Kritz

et al., 2009). Hser (2007) found no association between age and recovery. Similarly, treatment studies have reported that age does not predict abstinence (Darke *et al.*, 2005c, 2007d, 2009c; Kritz *et al.*, 2009). These data are consistent with the treatment outcome studies discussed in the previous chapter. It will be recalled that, when discussing predictors of treatment outcome, age was not mentioned. This was because it has not been demonstrated to be a relevant variable. It was individual factors such as heavier heroin and/or polydrug use, criminal involvement and some forms of psychopathology that predict drug status outcomes, not age. Indeed, two recent studies examining age and risk reported that older longer-term users displayed the same use patterns and levels of risk as their younger counterparts (Darke *et al.*, 2009c; Degenhardt *et al.*, 2008). In the former study, length of career was unrelated to heroin use, polydrug use, overdose, criminality or imprisonment. Users with careers in excess of 15 years exhibited the same use patterns and risk as those in the first 5 years of their trajectory.

Overall, there is little evidence to support the concept of maturing out of heroin dependence. While it may well have been a reasonable description of heroin use in the late 1950s and early 1960s (although this is questionable), it does not accord well with the trajectories seen since the heroin epidemics from the late 1960s onwards, and the cultural and cohort changes that were contiguous with these changes. This is not to say that all users who survive will continue to use. Certainly, some users *do* cease use relatively early. Remission rates for heroin dependence, however, are approximately half those of illicits such as the psychostimulants and cannabis (Calabria *et al.*, 2010). The predominant pattern is one of long-term dependent use that extends into the fifth and sixth decades of life. If such people are still to 'mature out', they have precious little time left in which to do so. Indeed, it is not at all clear what maturing out could possibly mean for people aged in their 40s, 50s and 60s.

Our hypothetical user thus has an excellent chance of still being a dependent user well past the age of 40. Such is the longevity of heroin use that the issue of aged care for heroin users is soon to become a major public health issue. Rather than mature out, we may see the advent of opioid maintenance within the parameters of nursing homes and hostels (Goldberg & Grabowski, 2003). Indeed, we are already seeing this (City of Vancouver, 2008; Judd, 2009). Elderly, opioid-maintained patients are highly likely to pose new and difficult challenges for these residential care facilities.

7.4   Morbidity and the older heroin user

We have established that large proportions of heroin users will use the drug in their 40s and beyond. We will now examine the physical and psychological morbidity associated with older heroin users. This remains a relatively unexplored area. The paucity of studies probably reflects the community focus on the stereotypical at risk young person, and the hidden assumption that drug use is a young person's problem. Old lives at risk do not carry the same cultural gravity as young lives at risk. The issue of old, long-term users is simply not 'sexy' to the general public and media. The lack of research may also reflect the fact that older users are only now appearing in large numbers. We will commence by examining issues surrounding physical morbidity in older users.

7.4.1   Physical morbidity

As discussed earlier, the physical health of the mature heroin user is typically poor, far poorer than that of non-users. At least some of this morbidity results from long-term infections such as HCV, which might well be expected to progress with age. The questions here are what clinically significant health problems are present in the older user, what organ systems do they manifest in and are the health problems of the older user worse than their younger counterparts? We must bear in mind that we are not talking about elderly people, who would be expected to have very high rates of health problems. Rather, it is people in their 40s and 50s we are addressing.

A number of studies have compared the global health of older heroin users to the general population, and to younger heroin users (Darke *et al.*, 2009c; Firoz & Carlson, 2004; Hser *et al.*, 2004; Lofwall *et al.*, 2005; Rajaratnam *et al.*, 2009; Rosen *et al.*, 2008). Both Rosen *et al.* (2008) and Hser *et al.* (2004) reported that older users had poorer health than the national average, controlling for sex and age. Of particular note, however, Rosen *et al.* (2008) found that, while the health of their group of 50–54-year-old users was poorer than non-users from the same age group, it was also poorer than non-users in the 55–67-year-old age group. Consistent with this, the authors noted that the physical health problems of these older users, such as arthritis and hypertension, were typical of much older age groups. Similarly, Lofwall *et al.* (2005) reported that older users had poorer health compared to non-users of the same age, than did younger users compared to their non-using peers. The general pattern appears to be one of accelerated ageing.

The few studies that have compared the health of older and younger users report that the health of the older user is significantly poorer than their younger counterparts (Clausen *et al.*, 2009; Darke *et al.*, 2009c; Firoz & Carlson, 2004; Lofwall *et al.*, 2005; Rajaratnam *et al.*, 2009). Lofwall *et al.* (2005) reported that older users had higher severity on global health and experienced significantly more sick days. Both Rajaratnam *et al.* (2009) and Firoz & Carlson (2004) reported that older users had higher levels of chronic medical problems. Indeed, the rate of chronic problems amongst older users in the Firoz & Carlson (2004) study was twice that of their younger counterparts. Consistent with these studies, Darke *et al.* (2009c) reported that the odds of severe physical disability increased 5% for each extra year of heroin use. Finally, pre-existing systemic disease amongst fatal overdose cases is also relevant, with age being a significant predictor of pre-existing cardiac, hepatic, pulmonary, renal and multiple system disease (Darke *et al.*, 2006a, 2010a). Consistent with this study, somatic causes of death increase in prevalence with age (Clausen *et al.*, 2009). In the Clausen *et al.* (2009) study, those over 50 were five times more likely to die from somatic causes than those younger than this, in which overdose plays a far more significant role. To summarise, older users are in poorer health than the general population and their younger counterparts. Moreover, the gap between the health of heroin users and others appears to widen with age.

We will now examine the different types of organ pathology seen amongst older heroin users. We will commence with the liver. Two points need to be made here. Firstly, in the general population the overall metabolic capacity of the liver is reduced in the elderly, due to factors such as decreases in liver mass, hepatic enzyme activity and hepatic blood flow (Schmucker, 2005). Secondly, it will be recalled that rates of HCV are extraordinarily high amongst heroin users, and may lead to hepatic cirrhosis, liver failure and hepatic carcinoma. Of course, the use of alcohol will exacerbate pathology and hasten disease progression. In addition, as we have already noted, morphine enhances HCV viral replication, and thus disease progression (Li *et al.*, 2007). As would be expected, the limited data indicate high levels of hepatic disease amongst the older user. Rosen *et al.* (2008) reported that 14% of their sample of methadone patients had cirrhotic livers, a progressive, degenerative disease that ends in liver failure and death. Amongst survivors of a similar age in the Hser *et al.* (2004) cohort, half had abnormal liver function. As discussed above, fatalities amongst heroin users provide information of relevance here (Darke *et al.*, 2006a). Amongst fatal heroin overdose cases, a quarter aged over 44 years had cirrhotic livers, compared to less than 5% of younger age groups (Darke *et al.*, 2006a). What should be borne in mind is that these people would have died from liver failure if they had not succumbed to overdose.

Clinically significant pulmonary disease also appears common amongst older users (Buster *et al.*, 2002; Darke *et al.*, 2006a; Hser *et al.*, 2004; Rosen *et al.*, 2008). This perhaps should not surprise. We have noted that one of the most consistent behavioural traits of heroin users is that they almost all smoke cigarettes (Hser *et al.*, 2004; McCool & Richter, 2003; Ross *et al.*, 2005). Long-term users are thus vulnerable to the harms associated with long-term tobacco consumption. One in five older users in Rosen *et al.* (2008) had chronic lung disease, and a third of the Hser *et al.* (2004) cohort had abnormal pulmonary functioning that indicated chronic obstructive lung disease. A similar result was seen in Buster *et al.* (2002). Amongst overdose fatalities, emphysema was present in 13% of cases aged over 44 years, compared to only 2% of younger cases (Darke *et al.*, 2006a). A similar result was also true for pulmonary fibrosis. Overall, the pulmonary health of the older users appears to be very poor.

Lifelong smoking also has cardiovascular implications, and older heroin users show high rates of cardiovascular pathology (Darke *et al.*, 2006a; Firoz & Carlson, 2004; Hser *et al.*, 2004; Lofwall *et al.*, 2005; Rosen *et al.*, 2008). More than half of the older users in Rosen *et al.* (2008) were diagnosed with hypertension, and a fifth had been diagnosed with some form of cardiac disease. Similarly, a half of the Hser *et al.* (2004) cohort were diagnosed with hypertension. Lofwall *et al.* (2005) reported that older users had far higher rates of cardiovascular disease compared to younger users (54% vs. 15%), with hypertension being the most common presentation (51% vs. 4%). As can be seen, the magnitude of the difference between older users and others is marked. To return once again to older overdose fatalities, one in five were diagnosed with severe coronary artery atherosclerosis and one in ten with ventricular hypertrophy (Darke *et al.*, 2006a). Furthermore, the rate of these pathologies increased monotonically with age. Thus, while a fifth of the older users had severe atherosclerosis, *none* of those aged under 25 exhibited this pathology.

We noted in an earlier chapter that the diet of the entrenched heroin user is very poor, with high intakes of sugar and fat. While the fat intake has cardiovascular implications for atherosclerotic vascular occlusion, the high sugar intake may engender Type II diabetes amongst older users. Both Rosen *et al.* (2008) and Hser *et al.* (2004) report that one in ten older users were diabetic. The fact that almost all heroin users smoke has serious implications for the diabetic user. Smoking is strongly counter-indicated for individuals suffering from diabetes, with increased risk of peripheral neuropathy and possible amputations due to restricted peripheral blood flow.

The apparent pattern of accelerated ageing seen amongst older users is also seen in their rates of arthritis (Lofwall *et al.*, 2005; Rosen *et al.*, 2008). In both these studies, over half of older users were arthritic, compared to one in five amongst younger users. The rates of degenerative bone disease seen in these studies amongst users in their 50s are more typical of a far older population than these middle-aged users.

Finally, an age-related health issue that is often overlooked, vascular health, should be briefly discussed. As we noted earlier, the very act of injecting causes vascular damage. As the use career progresses, injection sites become scarred and there is risk of vascular collapse. Indeed, some of the major health complaints of the older user are collapsed veins and abscesses on injection sites (Beynon *et al.*, 2009; Boeri *et al.*, 2008). Such damage is exacerbated if the user is an injector of oral preparations such as methadone syrup or benzodiazepines. As we noted in Chapter 5, there is a progression of injecting sites from the cubital fossa to more dangerous sites such as the neck and groin, and small veins in the hands and feet (Darke *et al.*, 2001b; Hoda *et al.*, 2008). In our study of injecting sites, we reported that injection universally commenced with the cubital fossa, with injections of the hand, neck and foot commencing approximately 5 years after initiation. Highly dangerous sites such as the groin were first accessed on average 10 years into the injecting career. Overall, it is highly likely that the older user, with a history of high intensity injecting, will have substantial vascular damage, and will be likely to use less accessible, and more dangerous, injection sites.

7.4.2 Psychopathology

The picture presented above in relation to physical morbidity is one of deterioration, reflecting disease progression and the effects of prolonged drug use. Is this the case for psychopathology? As we have discussed earlier, rates of psychopathology are extraordinarily high amongst mature heroin users. Does this pathology ameliorate or deteriorate with age? Unlike physical morbidity, the general picture of psychopathology appears to be one of stability. By this, I do not mean stable psychological functioning, but stable, high rates of psychopathology. Like physical health, however, the area is under-researched. The few studies that have been done, however, tell a consistent story. Rosen *et al.* (2008) reported that, amongst methadone patients aged over 50, over half had a current psychiatric disorder, with major depression (33%), generalised anxiety disorder (30%) and PTSD (28%) being the most prevalent diagnoses. By contrast, population rates for current diagnoses of major depression are approximately 2%–10%, 3% for generalised anxiety disorder and 8% for PTSD (APA, 2000). Our older user is experiencing a burden of disease that is still far in excess of population norms. On these figures, there appears to have been no improvements in mental health of the long-term user.

Several studies have compared rates of psychiatric morbidity of older and younger heroin users (Darke *et al.*, 2009c; Degenhardt *et al.*, 2008; Firoz & Carlson, 2004; Hser *et al.*, 2007a; Lofwall *et al.*, 2005). Firoz & Carlson (2004) found no difference in the prevalence of psychiatric problems, or their severity, between older and younger methadone patients. Lofwall *et al.* (2005) found no differences between older and younger maintenance patients in mood disorders, anxiety disorders or psychosis. Darke *et al.* (2009c) reported that length of career was not associated with severe psychiatric disability or a diagnosis of major depression. Finally, Degenhardt *et al.* (2008) found no differences in current mental health problems, or in mental health consultations, between groups aged under 25, 25–34, and 35 and older.

Consistent with the maintenance of high levels of pathology amongst long-term users, Hser *et al.* (2007a) reported that 'early quitters' showed lower rates of pathology than those who exhibited the dominant career trajectory of long-term, heavy use. This is consistent with the earlier conversation about the improvements in psychopathology that are associated with successful drug treatment. It would seem that, if the user maintains their use, they will continue to have high rates of distress. Indeed, qualitative research points to the fact that long-term heroin users find the lifestyle depressing (Beynon *et al.*, 2009; Hartel *et al.*, 2006). As we noted in Chapter 5, it is a hard life with a great deal of exposure to violence, unemployment, disease and death. In addition, users speak of increasing social isolation with advancing age. We must also keep in mind the high death rates amongst users, which we will explore in detail in the ensuing chapter. A long-term user will typically have lost many of their cohort to overdose, suicide, disease or trauma. We should also bear in mind the poor, and deteriorating, physical health of the older user. This is a group of sick, marginalised, socially isolated people. That they continue to be distressed should come as no great surprise.

7.5 Mortality risk and the older heroin user

Premature mortality is a major clinical issue for heroin users, and will be discussed in full in the next chapter. We will now, however, very briefly examine some of the implications of ageing for mortality and the older user. Independent of direct disease sequelae, the poor physical health of older users may place them at greater risk of heroin overdose. As we have seen, there is significant hepatic disease amongst older users, which has implications for drug metabolism. Slower metabolism, due to hepatic fibrosis or cirrhosis, may place the user at risk of overdose, and over greater periods of time, than the younger user. The obstructive lung disease seen in older users is also of potential clinical importance. Compromised lung function in the presence of a CNS depressant, such as heroin, may increase the risk of hypoxia and death following administration. The risk of cardiac arrest due to oxygen deprivation may also be exacerbated by pre-existing cardiovascular pathology. It should be noted in passing that these risks appears to be exacerbated in the presence of long-acting opioids such as methadone (Darke *et al.*, 2010a).

As discussed in Chapter 5, psychostimulant use is common amongst primary heroin users, drugs known to be cardiotoxic, and to place heavy demands upon the cardiovascular system. The higher level of cardiovascular pathology seen in the older heroin user is of concern here, as it may increase the risk of cardiovascular and cerebrovascular events.

The persistence of major psychiatric pathology across decades places older users at extended risk for suicide. The longer the exposure to these risk factors, the more likely the event is to occur. Furthermore, there are bimodal age-related peaks in the incidence of completed and attempted suicide, with an early peak late in the teens and early 20s, followed by a later life peak after the 50s. As the user moves to a higher risk demographic, the maintenance of use, and associated psychopathology, places them at considerable risk for suicide.

7.6 Summary

It is clear that many users will be using heroin well into middle age, and beyond. The hope that most users will mature out appears utterly misplaced. Rather, most will not do so, and will carry extraordinary burdens of physical and psychological disease across decades, if they survive. In our next chapter we will look at death amongst heroin users. Given all we have seen to date, this is a topic that is of great salience to heroin users, and those around them, and it all too frequently comes early.

Key points: Summary of the older heroin user: the 40s and beyond

- The 'maturing out' hypothesis is applied to the concept of heroin addicts outgrowing their drug habits, typically between the mid-20s and mid-30s.
- Support for the maturation hypothesis appears restricted to studies of users in the early 1960s, representing a cohort of users from the 1950s. Since then, the evidence for maturation is scant, with use into the fifth and sixth decades of life being common.
- Age and length of use career are *not* predictors of treatment outcome.
- Older heroin users are in poorer health than both the general population and their younger heroin using counterparts. Moreover, the gap between the health of heroin users and non-users widens with age.
- Older users have rates of hepatic, cardiovascular, pulmonary and musculoskeletal pathology that are more typical of the elderly.
- Psychiatric morbidity remains at extremely high levels. Unlike physical morbidity, there is no evidence of deterioration of psychopathology with age.
- The disease progression of the older user places them at greater risk of death from disease, overdose and suicide.

8

Death: rates and causes

8.1 Introduction

We come now to the end of life for our heroin user. Given all we have seen to date, it will not surprise the reader that death comes relatively early for many heroin users. Of course, not all heroin users will die an early, or even a drug-related, death. A great many, however, will. Indeed, as we discussed earlier, we would expect half to be deceased by the age of 50. The main causes of premature death amongst heroin users fall into four main areas: overdose, disease, suicide and trauma. Prior to exploring these causes, we must first examine death rates amongst heroin users, and how these relate to age and gender.

8.2 Rates of mortality

Longitudinal studies indicate mortality rates of 1% to 3% per annum, with mortality risk elevated by more frequent use (Bjornas *et al.*, 2008; Darke *et al.*, in press b; Gossop *et al.*, 2002b; Miller *et al.*, 2007; Smyth *et al.*, 2007; Stenbacka *et al.*, 2010). While these figures do not sound particularly high, in the majority of studies the mortality rate is at least ten times that of non-drug users. Consistent with the pattern of accelerated ageing we noted in the previous chapter, death rates amongst heroin users are more typical of a far older age group.

While studies from all countries show elevated death rates, those amongst heroin users in Asia are approximately twice those of western Europe, three times those of North America, and five times those of Australasia (Azim *et al.*, 2008; Degenhardt *et al.*, 2009b, 2011; Fugelstad *et al.*, 2007; Miller *et al.*, 2007; Quan *et al.*, 2007; Vlakov *et al.*, 2008; Zhang *et al.*, 2005). This in part reflects differences in underlying regional population mortality rates, but it may well also reflect differences in access to treatment and health care.

111

Two other factors also have strong influences upon mortality. Firstly, consistent with the reductions in drug use, enrolment in long-term treatment is associated with substantially reduced death rates (Clausen *et al.*, 2008, 2009; Degenhardt *et al.*, 2011; Scherbaum *et al.*, 2002; Soyka *et al.*, 2006). Indeed, mortality rates for those out of treatment are three to five times higher than those in treatment. Such is the strength of this effect that it has been estimated that long-term treatment adds an extra 20 years of life for a heroin user (Smyth *et al.*, 2007). As we have seen, long-term treatment reduces drug use frequency, risk-taking, criminality and rates of overdose, as well as improving global health, all of which dispose to reduced mortality rates. The second factor is route of administration. As we discussed earlier, non-injecting routes of administration are associated with lower risks for heroin overdose, blood-borne viruses, vascular damage and suicide, which translates directly into reduced mortality (Bird, 2010). Indeed, the higher the proportion of non-injectors in a cohort, the lower the mortality (Degenhardt *et al.*, 2011). The point needs to be reiterated, however, that whilst the overwhelming majority of overdose deaths are due to injecting heroin, cases of overdose via other routes have been documented (Darke & Ross, 2000).

The question arises as to whether heroin use is more risky than the use of other drugs, or are the high mortality rates merely a reflection of drug dependence *per se*? The former appears to be the case: heroin use carries a far greater risk of death than the regular use of other commonly abused drugs, such as methamphetamine. The few longitudinal studies that have addressed this issue consistently report significantly higher death rates amongst primary heroin users (Bartu *et al.*, 2004; Stenbacka *et al.*, 2010; Wahren *et al.*, 1997).

8.3   The demography of death amongst heroin users

8.3.1   Age and mortality

It is a common misconception in the public press that heroin-related deaths occur amongst the young. This is most certainly not the case, as the mean age at death of heroin users is consistently in the late 20s and early 30s (e.g. Darke *et al.*, 2010a; Degenhardt *et al.*, 2011). While deaths amongst younger users do occur, these are uncommon, and it is the older, experienced user who is at the greatest risk. Consistent with this, older age is repeatedly reported as an independent predictor of death (Bartu *et al.*, 2004; Brugal *et al.*, 2005; Degenhardt *et al.*, 2011; Gossop *et al.*, 2002b; Stenbacka *et al.*, 2010). While this is in one sense quiet prosaic (i.e. age will kill you in the end) it must be borne in mind that these are *not* elderly people.

A related, but not identical, variable of importance is the length of the heroin use career. A longer career has repeatedly been related to a higher risk of mortality (Brugal *et al.*, 2005; Hser *et al.*, 2001; Quaglio *et al.*, 2001; Vlahov *et al.*, 2004). Again, it is not the new user who is at greatest risk, but the established user. As we know, our typical heroin user commenced their use in their mid to late teens. The age at death suggests that they have typically been using illicit drugs for a decade or more when they die. Why this is the case will be addressed below.

8.3.2 Gender and mortality

The majority of deaths worldwide attributable to heroin use occur amongst males (Darke *et al.*, 2007a; Degenhardt *et al.*, 2011). Indeed, males constitute approximately three-quarters of deaths in both cohort and coronial studies. To an extent this reflects the epidemiology of heroin use, as we have seen that males comprise the bulk of heroin users. This does not mean, however, that the female heroin user is at less risk of death once she enters the world of heroin dependence. When gender specific mortality rates have been reported there is little, if any, difference between male and female death rates (Bargagli *et al.*, 2001, 2006; Bartu *et al.*, 2003; Darke *et al.*, 2010a, in press b; Goldstein & Herrara, 1995; Gossop *et al.*, 2002b; Orti *et al.*, 1996; Sanchez-Carbonell & Seus, 2000; Stenbacka *et al.*, 2010).

An issue that causes some confusion about comparative mortality rates is that the standardised mortality ratios (SMRs) associated with female mortality are generally greater than those of males (Bargagli *et al.*, 2001; Davoli *et al.*, 1997; Goldstein & Herrera, 1995; Rehm *et al.*, 2005; Stenbacka *et al.*, 2010). Thus, female heroin users are substantially more likely to die compared to other females, than males are when compared to other males. Does this mean that women heroin users are at greater risk than their male counterparts? Not in my opinion. While it is possible that female users are more risky than their male counterparts, the fact that their death rates are similar argues against such an interpretation. The more likely explanation is that there is a substantially lower base population mortality rate amongst females. If the mortality rates of male and female heroin users are similar, which they are, the SMRs of female drug users will be far greater. While the chances of death may be similar for both male and female drug users, the excess risk faced by females compared to their non-drug using female peers is substantially greater than that seen among males.

8.4   Causes of death

8.4.1   Overdose

Overdose is the most common cause of premature death for heroin users. This is perhaps not surprising, as there is a risk of an overdose associated with every use episode. The risk is immediate and consistent. Rates of non-fatal overdose discussed earlier clearly demonstrate this risk. The proportion of deaths attributable to overdose in major studies is approximately half, but has ranged from a quarter to over 80% (Antolini *et al.*, 2006; Bargagli *et al.*, 2001; Bartu *et al.*, 2004; Darke *et al.*, in press b; Degenhardt *et al.*, 2011; Hser *et al.*, 2001; Maxwell *et al.*, 2005; Odegard *et al.*, 2007; Oppenheimer *et al.*, 1994; Soyka *et al.*, 2006). The primary mechanism of death is heroin-induced respiratory depression, resulting in hypoxia and death (White & Irvine, 1999). Death from other opioids such as methadone, buprenorphine or oxycodone, also results from respiratory depression. The cardinal signs of heroin toxicity are reduced level of consciousness, pinpoint pupils and a depressed respiratory rate. Cyanosis, hypotension, bradycardia and hypothermia may also be present (Karch, 2009; White & Irvine, 1999).

The term 'overdose' is somewhat misleading. One of the great puzzles surrounding overdose is that morphine concentrations in fatalities are moderate in many cases (cf. Darke *et al.*, 2007a). Indeed, direct comparisons indicate that fatal overdose cases are likely to have morphine levels no higher than survivors or living intoxicated heroin users (Aderjan *et al.*, 1995; Darke *et al.*, 1997; Gutierrez-Cebollada *et al.*, 1994). Why this should be the case will be pursued below. Prior to this, we must first examine two common misconceptions that have been used to explain overdose, excess purity ('killer heroin') and contaminants (it is not the heroin, but what it is cut with). Firstly, fluctuations in heroin purity appear to have, at best, a moderate relationship to the incidence of heroin-related death, a fact first demonstrated in the 1970s (Darke *et al.*, 1999a; Desmond *et al.*, 1978; Risser *et al.*, 2000; Ruttenber & Luke, 1984). Secondly, harmful contaminants are rarely detected, and are typically innocuous substances, such as sucrose (Coomber, 1999; Maher *et al.*, 2001). There is no toxicological evidence that contaminants play a major role in heroin overdose.

What then is the real toxicological picture of overdose? The most important finding to emerge in research regarding overdose is that the majority of cases involve the concomitant consumption of other drugs, of which alcohol and benzodiazepines are the most important (Darke *et al.*, 2010a; Davidson *et al.*,

2003; Fugelstad *et al.*, 2003; Hickman *et al.*, 2003; Preti *et al.*, 2002). Importantly, concomitant polydrug use also extends to deaths attributed to other opioids, such methadone, buprenorphine and oxycodone (Boyd *et al.*, 2003; Bryant *et al.*, 2003; Darke *et al.*, 2010a; Hickman *et al.*, 2003; Seymour *et al.*, 2003).

In light of the polydrug use of heroin users, the fact that multiple drugs are found is not surprising. These are not, however, mere artefacts, but play a direct role in these deaths. Co-administration of other depressant drugs substantially increases the likelihood of a fatal outcome due to the potentiation of the respiratory depressant effects of heroin. In the presence of CNS depressants, the usual dose of heroin may well prove fatal. By far the most common drug detected is alcohol, present in half or more of cases (Darke *et al.*, 2010a; Davidson *et al.*, 2003; Fugelstad *et al.*, 2003; Hickman *et al.*, 2003; Preti *et al.*, 2002). There is an inverse relationship between blood morphine and alcohol concentrations, with lower morphine concentrations detected in the presence of alcohol (Darke *et al.*, 2000; Fugelstad *et al.*, 2003; Ruttenber *et al.*, 1990; Ruttenber & Luke, 1984). Benzodiazepines are noted in up to quarter of cases, and have been shown to decrease oxygen saturation substantially in conjunction with opioids (Darke *et al.*, 2010a; Davidson *et al.*, 2003; Fugelstad *et al.*, 2003; Lintzeros *et al.*, 2006, 2007). In fact, there is evidence of an increase in the frequency of benzodiazepine prescriptions in the weeks preceding death (Burns *et al.*, 2004; Martyres *et al.*, 2004). The presence of CNS depressants in overdose provides a possible explanation of the surprisingly low morphine concentrations seen in many overdose deaths. These are multiple drug toxicity deaths, in which each individual substance may well be present in sub-toxic concentrations.

The concomitant use of psychostimulants is also relevant. As we have seen, psychostimulants place heavy demands upon the cardiovascular system through increased heart rate, blood pressure and myocardial oxygen demand. Heroin, in contrast, depresses respiration. The combination of heroin and a psychostimulant may thus produce a situation in which there is increased myocardial oxygen demand with a contiguous depression of respiration. It may further be speculated that respiratory depression may induce cardiac failure, particularly among people where cardiac disease is present.

There are several possible reasons why the typical overdose case is around 30 years old. Each use episode carries a risk of overdose, and the cumulative risk may be such that the risk of death is substantially higher at 30 than at 18. It will also be recalled that the first overdose usually occurs after a couple of years of use, and after the development of dependence, so fewer young cases would be expected. The natural history of heroin tolerance may also partially explain the phenomenon. It has been suggested that tolerance to the hedonistic effects of opioids develops more rapidly than to the respiratory effects, with the latter being an incomplete tolerance (White & Irvine, 1999). As the use career progresses, the gap between the dose needed to obtain a hedonistic effect and the lethal dose decreases. Given this, it is longer-term heroin users who would be most likely to suffer overdoses.

There are specific situations in which tolerance plays a major role. In particular, the period immediately post-prison release, or after the cessation of treatment constitute high risk periods for fatal overdose (Davoli *et al.*, 2007; Farrell & Marsden, 2008; Ravndal & Amundsen, 2010; Seymour *et al.*, 2003). Similar transient risks exist when heroin use resumes after maintenance on the opioid antagonist naltrexone, and in the period immediately following a successful opioid detoxification (Digiusto *et al.*, 2004; Miotto *et al.*, 1997; Oliver *et al.*, 2005; Strang *et al.*, 2003).

An alternative, though not incompatible, explanation of the age demographic relates to the natural history of heroin use itself. Recent studies have reported that hair morphine concentrations among fatal overdose cases are significantly lower than those of current users, indicating less frequent heroin use among many users in the period immediately preceding death (Darke *et al.*, 2002a; Fugeslstad *et al.*, 2003; Kronstrand *et al.*, 1998; Tagliaro *et al.*, 1998). The rigours of the heroin lifestyle may mean that, after a decade or so of heroin use, many users cut down their use. They may also increase their use of other drugs, such as alcohol and benzodiazepines, to compensate for their reduced heroin use. Finally, it is possible that underlying systemic disease progression amongst older users may affect their ability to metabolise drugs.

An excess of male overdose cases is not surprising, given their over-representation among heroin users. Whilst males represent approximately two-thirds of opiate users, however, they constitute substantially higher proportions of fatalities. Two possible explanatory factors are the higher rates of alcohol use of males, and their greater social isolation. Male heroin users are more likely to be alcohol dependent than females, and are more likely to have alcohol detected in overdose fatalities (Darke *et al.*, 2007a). They are also less likely to be married, or to live with others and as such, are more likely to be alone at the time of an overdose (Davoli *et al.*, 1993).

8.4.2 Disease

Disease is one of the major killers of heroin users (Darke *et al.*, 2007a). Along with the epidemiology of overdose, the disease process may also explain the relatively 'old' mean age of death seen in cohort studies. By definition, disease progression will correlate with older age, particularly the long-term sequelae of HIV or HCV infection. Older users may thus be sicker, and die due to illness. Indeed, the pattern of accelerated ageing of heroin users is consistent with this scenario.

In most studies since the late 1970s (after the advent of the HIV pandemic), deaths due to disease, most commonly acquired immunodeficiency syndrome (AIDS), have ranged from 30% to over 70% (Bargagli *et al.*, 2001, 2006; Bartu *et al.*, 2004; Degenhardt *et al.*, 2011; Gossop *et al.*, 2002b; Manfredi *et al.*, 2006; Maxwell *et al.*, 2005; Rehm *et al.*, 2005; Sanchez-Carbonell & Seus, 2000). It is clear that disease poses a major threat to heroin users. Moreover, HIV positive drug users die at even greater rates than the high rates of the HIV negative user, due to both AIDS and other causes (Degenhardt *et al.*, 2011; Tyndall *et al.*, 2001).

Cause of death amongst heroin users (and IDU more generally) show considerable temporal variations. While AIDS has remained a major cause of death amongst heroin users, since the 1990s there appear to have been decreases in AIDS-related mortality, even in high seroprevalence countries, that have coincided with the advent of highly active antiretroviral therapies (Bargagli *et al.*, 2006; Degenhardt *et al.*, 2011; Vlahov *et al.*, 2005). In high seroprevalence Italy, for instance, AIDS supplanted overdose as the major cause of death amongst heroin users in the late 1980s, but overdose reasserted its role in the late 1990s (Davoli *et al.*, 1997).

Sexual transmission of HIV is a significant factor for heroin users. In high seroprevalence countries, drug users with more sexual partners are more likely to be HIV positive (Doherty *et al.*, 2000). As we know, many heroin users engage in sex work to support their use, which places them at greater risk of contracting HIV, particularly if they are engaging in highly risky sexual behaviours.

The prevalence of HCV among IDU is much higher than that of HIV. To date, mortality related to HCV has been lower than HIV (Degenhardt *et al.*, 2011; Karch, 2009). This may change as IDU who have chronic HCV infections age, and develop liver cirrhosis and end-stage liver disease.

In concluding, it is important to note that, while the pathologies discussed above are the diseases of most relevance to heroin users, there is increased risk of death across all forms of disease. This reflects the role of viruses such as HIV, and the generally poor health of heroin users.

8.4.3   Suicide

While it is a relatively neglected area of research in the drug and alcohol field, suicide is a major cause of death amongst heroin users. It is estimated that heroin dependence is associated with a completed suicide risk 14 times that of the general population (Harris & Barraclough, 1997; Wilcox *et al.*, 2004). The impact of drug dependence upon suicide at a population level is seen in the high rates of opioids present in the blood of completed suicides (Darke *et al.*, 2009a; Dhosshe *et al.*, 2001; Shields *et al.*, 2006). In a recent study of violent (non-poisoning) completed suicides, opioids were present at over 40 times the level expected from population use figures (Darke *et al.*, 2009a).

To understand why rates of completed suicide are so high amongst heroin users, we need to examine the risk factors for suicide. These risk factors fall into four broad areas: demographics, psychopathology, family dysfunction and social isolation/dysfunction. One of the outstanding features of these risk factors is that they are almost a redescription of heroin users. Regular, dependent users have an extremely high prevalence for all these risk factors, and these factors have been associated specifically with suicide risk among heroin users (Darke & Ross, 2002; Johnsson & Fridell, 1997; Rossow & Lauritzen, 2001; Roy, 2010).

Males form the bulk of completed suicides, being three times more likely to complete than females (Bertelote & Fleischmann, 2002; Diekstra, 1996). Suicide is particularly prevalent amongst the young, with suicide rates being highest amongst teenagers and those aged in their 20s (Bertelote & Fleischmann, 2002; Diekstra, 1996; Johnstone *et al.*, 2009; Lynskey *et al.*, 2000), ages that broadly correspond to those in which rates of heroin use are at their highest. Thus, apart from other risk factors, heroin users broadly lie in the age range in which suicidality is most common. It should be noted that the second demographic peak in suicide amongst the elderly may become of direct relevance to ageing heroin using cohorts. As we have seen, the psychopathology of the older heroin users remains high, while their physical heath deteriorates.

A range of psychopathology has been associated with suicide. Not surprisingly, mood disorders have a particularly strong relationship, with the risk increased 20-fold (Harris & Barraclough, 1997; Wilcox *et al.*, 2004). Anxiety disorders, including panic disorders and agoraphobia, are associated with a

6–12 times increased risk of completed suicide (Harris & Barraclough, 1997; Wilcox *et al.*, 2004). In particular, PTSD is strongly associated with suicide (APA, 2000). Personality disorders, as a group, have been related to attempted and completed suicide (APA, 2000; Wilcox *et al.*, 2004). BPD and CD in particular are associated with substantially elevated risk. As we have noted earlier, the rates of all these forms of psychopathology are substantially elevated amongst heroin users.

A history of family dysfunction or disadvantage strongly predicts suicidal behaviours, in particular low socioeconomic status, parental separation prior to age 15 and parental psychopathology (particularly depression). It is also known that a history of childhood sexual or physical abuse substantially increases the risk of suicide (Maloney *et al.*, 2009). As we have discussed, this is almost a redescription of the childhood experiences of many heroin users.

Not surprisingly, social isolation and disadvantage increase the risk of suicide (Appleby *et al.*, 1999; Bertelote & Fleischmann, 2002; Hassan, 1995). In particular, perceived lack of social support, unemployment and homelessness all heighten risk. What is of direct clinical relevance here is that, as with psychopathology and traumatising childhood experiences, this is almost a redescription of the heavily dependent heroin user. Given their widespread exposure to multiple suicide risk factors, it is not surprising that the rates of both completed and attempted suicide amongst illicit drug users are many times those of the general community.

Before closing this section on suicide, it is necessary to distinguish between suicide and overdose, which are frequently confounded. Whilst it must be accepted that there are problems differentiating deliberate and accidental overdose, most overdoses are accidental, and the toxicology of these two events differ (Darke *et al.*, 2010b). As would be expected, if they are different phenomena, they are also predicted by different factors. Thus, while suicide is predicted by factors such as mood disorder and social isolation, overdose is predicted by factors such as concomitant use of other CNS depressants and route of administration (Maloney *et al.*, 2009). Moreover, when asked if their overdoses were deliberate, almost all say no (Darke & Ross, 2001; Tobin & Latkin, 2003). Overall, heroin overdoses constitute only a small proportion of completed and attempted suicides amongst heroin users. Indeed, most illicit drug user suicides employ means other than their drug of dependence. Why this should be the case is intriguing. Drug users have access to their drug of choice, and in the case of heroin this is an obvious means of self-poisoning. It is possible that drug users associate their drug with pleasure, rather than a means of suicide.

8.4.4   Trauma

As has been reiterated throughout this book, the lifestyle of the dependent heroin user is filled with risk, including a high risk of traumatic injury. Given these levels of risk exposure, it would be expected that death due to trauma would constitute a significant proportion of heroin user deaths. This appears to be the case. The proportion of deaths, in cohort and coronial studies, attributable to trauma has ranged up to nearly half, with most studies reporting proportions in the 10%–20% range (Davoli *et al.*, 1997; Degenhardt *et al.*, 2011; Digiusto *et al.*, 2004; Goldstein & Herrera, 1995; Gossop *et al.*, 2002b; Oppenheimer *et al.*, 1994).

Firstly, and not surprisingly, homicide plays a significant role, with studies of heroin users reporting homicide fatalities in the 5%–15% range (cf. Darke *et al.*, 2007a). The role of heroin, and other illicit drugs, in homicide is demonstrated by findings that as many as a third of victims test positive for illicit drugs (Darke, 2010). Recent studies in the USA and Australia reported that approximately one in ten homicide victims were positive for opioids, more than 40 times what would be expected (Darke & Duflou, 2008; Tardiff *et al.*, 2005).

Traumatic death amongst our target population is not confined to homicide. Heroin users frequently drive whilst intoxicated (Aitken *et al.*, 2000; Albery *et al.*, 2000; Darke *et al.*, 2003a). Given the frequency of intoxicated driving by heroin and other illicit drug users, and the higher frequency of accidents, we would expect substance use to be a major contributor to motor vehicle accidents' (MVA) trauma (Kelly *et al.*, 2004). Such appears to be the case. Internationally, studies report alcohol in excess of legal limits in 10%–50% of fatal accidents, and of other drugs between 5% and 30% (cf. Kelly *et al.*, 2004). Consistent with the polydrug use of illicit drug users, multiple drug detection is common, and 5%–20% of killed or injured drivers have alcohol/ drug combinations detected. In most studies of mortality amongst heroin users, deaths due to road trauma comprises a substantial proportion of trauma fatalities (cf. Darke *et al.*, 2007a).

Finally, the impairments in psychomotor performance, alertness and judgement noted in relation to driving also have implications for accidents due to other causes. Impairment due to intoxication with heroin and other drugs may well increase the risk of fatal accidents due to falls from heights, drownings, etc. As with MVA and homicides, illicit drugs are commonly detected in non-MVA trauma victims (Gill, 2001; Gill & Catanese, 2002; Lucas *et al.*, 2002; Turk & Tsokos, 2004). By way of example, Turk & Tsokos (2004) reported one in ten accidental fatal falls from heights were positive for morphine or cocaine. Similarly, high proportions have been found for accidental drowning (Lucas *et al.*, 2002), occupational fatalities (Greenberg *et al.*, 1999) and accidental sharp object injuries (Gill & Catanese, 2002). The proportion of deaths caused by non-MVA trauma amongst heroin users is not often reported. Where it has been reported, the data suggest that non-MVA trauma plays a significant role in mortality, with rates comparable to deaths from MVA trauma (Darke *et al.*, 2007a).

8.5 Summary

In summary, death poses a major risk to the long-term heroin user. While it comes early to many, on average it does so after 10 or so years of heroin use. As can be seen in this chapter, the causes of premature death are not restricted to drug use (e.g. overdose), or to disease. Violence to the self and traumatic injury make large contributions to the burden of mortality, although they are less well recognised. In the next chapter we will examine whether premature death is a necessary end for heroin users, or at least for substantial proportions of this population. The question we must ask is whether we can change the trajectories to avoid this.

Key points: Summary of death: rates and causes

- Heroin users have an excess mortality rate approximately 13 times higher than their peers. We would expect half to be deceased by age 50.
- Death rates among heroin users vary considerably by geographic region, and are highest in Asia.
- Lower mortality rates are associated with being enrolled in long-term treatment, and non-injecting routes of administration.
- The average age at death is in the early 30s. There are few cases of death under the age of 20.
- Death rates are similar for males and females. Female heroin users, however, are substantially more likely to die compared to other females, than are males when compared to other males.
- The major causes of death are overdose, disease, suicide and trauma.

9

Conclusions: an inevitable life and death?

9.1 The lifecycle: a retrospective

We come now to the final chapter in our examination of the life trajectories of heroin users. In this chapter we will briefly examine the implications of what we know of typical trajectories for public health and clinical practice.

Before we proceed, let us first reiterate the major findings of the preceding chapters, as they will inform our considerations. Firstly, extremely high proportions, perhaps the majority, of heroin users were victims of sexual and/or physical abuse during childhood. Large proportions grow up in dysfunctional families where parental drug and alcohol abuse are common, as is the absence of parents. While clearly not true of everyone who is dependent, we are dealing with a group that, as a whole, carries a substantial burden of trauma prior to the onset of heroin dependence. Moreover, the use of heroin typically begins after initiation into other drugs such as alcohol and cannabis, setting up a persistent pattern of lifetime polydrug use.

The second point to note is the high dependence liability of heroin. As we noted, the dependence liability of heroin is second only to that of tobacco. We currently believe that around one in four who ever use heroin will become dependent upon it. The risk of a transition from any use to problematic use is thus extremely high. Furthermore, once dependence is established, the user is exposed to a range of serious health and drug-related problems that include overdose, psychiatric comorbidity, blood-borne viral infection, social isolation and an entrenchment in crime.

The third salient point here is the sheer chronicity of heroin dependence. As we learned, the remission rates for heroin dependence are half those of other illicit drugs (Calabria *et al.*, 2010). Rather than mature out, the predominant trajectory appears to be one of long-term dependence, with many active users now in their sixth decade or beyond. The health of those who continue to use and survive is extremely poor, with marked premature ageing.

Fourthly, in any trajectory, potentially significant turning points will occur. These may be conceptualised as 'opportunities' to deflect the trajectory towards reduced use and harm, or indeed to total abstinence. While such significant life turning points may be manifold, the two most salient are drug treatment enrolment and incarceration. These opportunities, if we may characterise them as such, tend to recur. There will very likely be multiple treatment enrolments, arrests and incarcerations.

Finally, as we saw in the previous chapter, the risk of mortality is extremely high. Indeed, the lethality of heroin dependence is higher than that of any other drug class.

9.2   Clinical implications

9.2.1   An inevitable trajectory?

The picture presented in this book of the long-term trajectory of the heroin user is rather bleak. Is this inevitable? Need a long-term spiral into dependence, disease and death always be the case? Can the 'career path' be altered, or if not, can the harm to the individual and society be reduced? Of course, we know that there is no one single trajectory. The work on long-term cohorts suggest that early quitters do exist. We are also aware of the existence of what Hser and colleagues referred to as 'decelerated' users, who may have careers of a decade or so, but then taper off (Hser *et al.*, 2007a). A decade of heroin use is still, however, a long time, filled with high risk. Stable high-level users who may use over the course of decades, interspersed with treatment and incarceration, however, exist in large numbers, and appear to constitute the dominant trajectory. Even if this is not so, the existence of users who have used over the course of three or more decades cannot be disputed. Given what we know about the high dependence liability of heroin, and the extensive childhood abuse and psychopathology of users, a prolonged trajectory is not surprising.

Quantum theory has taught us that nothing is inevitable. Rather, we live in a probabilistic universe. What then do we do to reduce heroin consumption, and reduce the extensive harms and costs of such consumption? Three broad approaches will be considered, which are in no way to be seen as mutually exclusive. Firstly, given the high dependence liability of heroin, we will consider strategies for preventing the uptake of heroin and other substances.

Secondly, we will discuss drug treatment, one of the major turning points in heroin trajectories. Within this framework, the potential for treatment within the prison system will also be briefly examined. Finally, given the chronicity of heroin dependence, and that that even 'decelerators' have prolonged use, we will examine ways of reducing the morbidity and mortality of heroin dependence that fall under the general rubric 'harm reduction'. These may be conceptualised as a range of measures designed to keep users alive and healthy, in recognition of the chronicity of dependence and the harm it causes to users and the community.

9.2.2 *Prevention*

The first approach we should consider is to avoid the start of the trajectory altogether, or at least to delay it. As we have seen, early onset is associated with greater harm, so a delay of the development of dependence may also have some benefits. A number of means can be considered here. The first, and probably most widely recognised by the general population, are community level drug awareness campaigns modelled upon social marketing principles. The aim here is to achieve desirable behavioural change at the community level, through mass marketing techniques that are used to provide information on the harms of a substance, and to make its use less attractive, or even unacceptable (Goren, 2005; Kotler & Zaltman, 1971). Such campaigns may be targeted at the whole community, such as television and billboard advertisements, or towards particular groups of drug users. Anti-smoking campaigns are probably the best-known template for broad community level approaches, and have contributed to the decline in smoking prevalence and social acceptability in many countries around the world.

Of course, in the case of tobacco smoking, the prevalence in the community was (and in many countries is still) extremely high. The target audience was thus large, and covered a wide demographic. The problem with heroin use is that it is a low prevalence behaviour, in the order of 2% of the population. For the vast majority of those to whom the material is displayed, it is simply not relevant.

Given that it is the young who have not yet commenced a heroin trajectory, a major prevention focus is school-based drug education (McBride, 2003; Newton *et al.*, 2009, 2010; Tobler & Stratton, 1997; Vogl *et al.*, 2009; White & Pitts, 1998). Such campaigns typically focus on improving the knowledge amongst school students of the harms associated with certain drugs, and delaying or preventing the onset of their use. Consistent with their epidemiology, the two substances most commonly addressed are alcohol and cannabis. As we have seen, it is a very unusual heroin user who commenced their drug use career with heroin. Rather, heroin use typically emerges after substantive earlier substance involvement. Reducing the risk of being enmeshed in substance use, and its culture, may well reduce the risk of commencing heroin use. Indeed, there is emerging evidence to suggest that school-based drug education may have a significant effect in preventing drug use among young people (Botvin & Griffin, 2007; Cuijpers, 2002, 2010; McBride, 2003; Newton *et al.*, 2009; Tobler & Stratton, 1997; Vogl *et al.*, 2009; White & Pitts, 1998). Recent work on a web-based intervention, for instance, demonstrated increases in knowledge of alcohol and cannabis across 12 months amongst 13-year-old high school students and, more importantly, reductions in alcohol consumption (Newton *et al.*, 2009, 2010; Vogl *et al.*, 2009). We are not specifically addressing the heroin use career here, but early involvement in substance use *per se*. Importantly, it makes no difference whether we accept the tenets of gateway theory or common factor models, as both predict a reduced probability for heroin dependence.

Of course, school is just one aspect of a young person's life. There is also evidence that family-based interventions may prevent early onset alcohol use and intoxication (Foxcroft *et al.*, 2003). A recent review concluded that family involvement with activities such as parenting skills, parental education about drugs and skills increasing parents' confidence in communicating with young people about drugs were important in preventing substance use among young people (Velleman *et al.*, 2005; Vimpani, 2005).

Overall, campaigns to prevent the move into substance use and the heroin trajectory appear well worth it. For many, however, the trajectory will begin, particularly those with the kinds of family backgrounds we discussed in Chapter 2. This leads us to the second area of intervention, treatment.

9.2.3 Treatment

The single most significant potential turning point in the trajectory is treatment enrolment. As we saw in Chapter 6, retention in the long-term treatment modalities is associated with substantial, and rapid, improvements in clinical profile. Long-term retention is associated with large reductions in heroin use, declines in polydrug use, as well as reduced rates of overdose, injecting and needle sharing. We also know that criminality declines, as it is primarily driven by the need to acquire illicit drugs, and that both psychological and physical health improve substantially. Finally, and most importantly, treatment is associated with substantially reduced death rates. Given the lethality of heroin, this is a paramount consideration. Two points need to be made about treatment. Firstly, it is cost-effective. In the UK, for instance, it is estimated that, for every pound spent on treatment, there were savings to the community of three pounds (Godfrey *et al.*, 2004). When we consider the direct and indirect costs of heroin addiction, this makes perfect sense. Medical costs, including ambulance callouts, decline, as do the costs of crime. Life expectancy increases, so productivity and consumption are also likely to increase. Overall, this seems to be an excellent investment. The second point to note is that treatment is the most politically acceptable intervention to ameliorate heroin dependence. While other types of interventions discussed below, such as sterile needle provision, always invite controversy, the expansion of treatment is far more palatable to the general public and politicians.

The major point to be made here is that heroin users are *not* untreatable. Users are not necessarily chained to a single trajectory. The reductions in crime are particularly illustrative. It is sometimes naïvely believed that heroin users are, essentially, sociopaths, whose crime and drug use are intractable. The fact that crime declines with heroin use gives the lie to this argument. We can make a difference. We must, however, be realistic in our expectations. As we have seen, it is extremely unlikely that a single treatment episode will result in complete recovery. Given the dependence liability of heroin, the lengthy histories of abuse and the chronicity of dependence, this should not surprise. We also know that users typically do not enter treatment until they have developed dependence and a constellation of serious and potentially life-threatening drug-related problems. Those who enter treatment generally do so when things are at their worst. These are distressed people, and we should not be surprised that relapse rates are high. Importantly, as we noted earlier, while rates of sustained abstinence are low, there is evidence that periods of prolonged abstinence increase over time (Darke *et al.*, 2007d). Furthermore, we must keep in mind the 'decelerators' discussed above, whose deceleration may be enhanced by treatment. Heroin may well have lower remission rates than other illicit substances, but people can, and do, remit. While some users will only achieve short-term gains whilst enrolled in treatment, which is certainly worthwhile, substantial long-term gains will be seen in many.

As we noted in Chapter 6, the major treatment modalities in the treatment cycle are detoxification, heroin maintenance and antagonist therapies and residential rehabilitation. Perhaps the most notable clinical implication to emerge from studies of treatment outcome is the importance of *stable retention*. Clinically, this may be extremely difficult, particularly with more dysfunctional clients. Furthermore, we know that it is precisely the more poorly functioning, drug-entrenched user who has the poorest prognosis. The chances of a successful outcome, even for such clients, improves dramatically the longer they can be retained in treatment. These are long-term problems that are likely to require long-term solutions. The 'serial enroller' may well be exposed to a great deal of treatment over time, but will not typically show the improvement of those retained over fewer treatment episodes.

The repeated finding that it is long-term retention that makes the substantial treatment impacts clearly illustrates the need for long-term treatment integration and stabilisation. It does not matter here whether we are talking about agonist maintenance treatments or drug-free residential rehabilitation. As noted earlier, there is sometimes an ideological tension between supporters of agonist maintenance and abstinence treatments. The argument against maintenance is that we are prescribing an opioid to a heroin user, which is considered morally wrong. Yes, we are indeed prescribing drugs to a drug user. In doing so, lives are saved. In my opinion, there is no coherent argument that can be raised against a treatment of known efficacy, sought by those who do not wish (or cannot achieve) complete abstinence, and that reduces the risk of disease and death. To withhold a treatment known to be effective, on the basis of some ideological nicety, appears to me a dereliction of the duty of care.

Similarly, some of the most ardent adherents of maintenance appear to denigrate abstinence treatments. Again, we should not take such views too seriously. The evidence is that long-term retention in therapeutic communities produces similar outcomes to maintenance treatments. As we noted, users will attend either type of treatment, depending on whether they are ready for an abstinence approach or not. It will be a great blessing for us all when polemicists from either side of this pointless debate take a lead from their clients. Everything we know about the developmental histories of users, the abuse liability of heroin and its remarkable chronicity, is consistent with the data on the need for long-term (and probably repeated) treatment. As we have seen, detoxification is a short-term intervention of around a week. While it may have appeal as a means of rapid intervention, the efficacy of detoxification for long-term outcomes is poor (Hubbard *et al.*, 1997). As I argued earlier, detoxification should *not* be seen as a treatment intervention in and of itself, but as a gateway to more extensive treatment. In my opinion anyone who says that they can 'cure' an addict with a detoxification, whether rapid, sleep-based or otherwise is selling snake-oil. Ironically, those who engage in detoxification as a standalone intervention may actually be at *greater* risk of overdose than if they had not detoxified at all.

Antagonist therapies, such as naltrexone maintenance, may also offer the hope of long-term retention. As noted in Chapter 6, however, to date, retention on naltrexone maintenance is poor, and poor compliance with drugs such as these has implications for overdose if relapse does occur. It is possible, however, that implantable depot formulations may improve retention and reduce overdose risk. Again, the point to note here is that it is long-term stable retention that is of importance, not the treatment modality. As with other modalities, there are proponents of naltrexone maintenance who appear to believe that it is the *only* treatment of choice. There is *no* single treatment of choice for heroin dependence. Current trends suggest that naltrexone maintenance will likely remain a minority modality in the suite of treatment options.

Finally, there are two points in the life course that appear to require improvements in our treatment provision. Firstly, there is a lag of some 5 to 10 years between the onset of problematic drug use and initial treatment seeking. Early intervention is good intervention. Making treatment more available, and palatable, to younger users would appear wise. It is here that we may have the greatest chance to alter long-term trajectories. At the other end of the life continuum, we have the problem of the geriatric user. As we saw in Chapter 7, there are increasing numbers of older users, who have followed the predominant trajectory of long-term dependence. These people are at particular risk, and in far poorer health than their younger colleagues, and non-using peers. Issues of geriatric medicine will become increasingly salient, particularly in terms of dosage for drugs such as methadone as physical decline accelerates. Methadone in the nursing home is already starting to appear (City of Vancouver, 2008; Judd, 2009). Given all we know of the longevity of dependence, this issue will become a major one in the coming decades.

Before leaving the issue of treatment, we should note that incarceration also represents a major potential turning point. This is important for two reasons. Firstly, it offers the possibility of treatment within the prison system, particularly maintenance treatments. Indeed, in a number of countries agonist maintenance treatment is available in prison (Dolan *et al.*, 2003, 2005). There is, literally, a captive audience for such interventions. We should keep in mind that heroin use *does* occur in prisons, and such use comes at extremely high risk of blood-borne viral infection and overdose. Moreover, as we noted earlier, the 2 weeks immediately post-prison release is associated with a substantially elevated risk of mortality, primarily due to overdose. Agonist maintenance during incarceration, transferring into the community upon release, would be expected to reduce the risk of a tolerance-related overdose, as well as reducing the chances of disease transmission whilst in prison.

The bottom line here is that long-term, stable treatment reduces drug use and reduces risk. It keeps people alive and in substantially better heath than they would otherwise be. Yes, they may still use whilst in treatment (although generally at reduced rates). Yes, they still die at higher rates than the general population. These are, after all, a very risky group. The reductions in drug use, morbidity and mortality that flow from treatment are, however, indisputable. Treatment may deflect a trajectory, and in doing so gives enormous cost benefits to society, as well as tangible and intangible benefits to the individual and their families.

9.2.4 *Harm reduction*

Finally, we come to the suite of non-treatment interventions that fall under the broad term '*harm reduction*'. It is important to note that these interventions are not antithetical to the provision of drug treatment, and may well provide useful adjuncts for reducing mortality and morbidity. The rationale for harm reduction measures lies in the chronicity of dependence, and the serious harms to the self and others that heroin (and other drug) dependence engenders. All that we have seen of trajectories in this book indicates that we must accept that, for many users, the career will be extremely long, and filled with risk. In this section we will examine a few of the major and most topical interventions, including needle and syringe programmes, overdose prevention and medically supervised injecting centres.

Before describing these interventions, and their rationales, we must first briefly examine the philosophical issues raised here. For reasons that mystify me, the term 'harm reduction' raises curious passions in many. The primary argument against such measures is that they inherently condone or enable drug use. In considering this issue, we must return to what we know of heroin use. Firstly, there is the high dependence liability. Secondly, the trajectory, despite all efforts to the contrary, is likely to be long. Thirdly, the user is exposed to a range of serious health and drug-related problems that not only affect them, but the broader community. The average user will continue to use heroin whether harm reduction measures exist or not. Indeed, they did so for decades prior to the implementation of such approaches in the 1980s. Given the recognition that use will continue to occur, making such use safer for the individual, and at less cost to society, appears logical. HIV, for instance, does not restrict itself to IDU, but can leap from this population to the broader community. Harm reduction measures should be viewed under the broader rubric of public health. Such measures attempt to reduce harm to the individual user, and thus reduce the overall burden of disease to society. Providers of such services do not condone drug use, but recognise its existence and chronicity. Such interventions also offer the hope of integration into the broader health system (and possibly drug treatment) for a particularly damaged and marginalised group. To suggest, for example, that providing sterile injecting equipment to an IDU is encouraging them to use drugs appears to me to be absurd. They will do so in any case, and they will simply cost society more through more unsafe practices.

9.2.4.1   Needle and syringe provision

The most widespread harm reduction measure aimed at IDU, whether heroin users or otherwise, is the provision of sterile injecting equipment. The rationale for this lies in the fact that many of the major health problems associated with injecting drug use are due to blood-borne infections. As we saw in previous chapters, blood-borne viruses such as HIV are major causes of poor health and premature death amongst IDU. As we know, one of the major transmission routes of HIV and the hepatitis viruses is the sharing of unsterile injecting equipment. Indeed, HCV is almost exclusively transmitted through this vector. Users who share equipment are also exposed to a range of other infections. While not a treatment, or an intervention aimed at achieving reduced use or abstinence, sterile needle provision may still be viewed as an attempt to affect the trajectory of the user. The aim is to prevent infection amongst users, to improve their general health and reduce the risk of transmission to the broader community. In terms of the costs discussed in Chapter 1, the aim is to reduce the costs of medical care associated with infection, as well as reduce mortality and DALYs. An uninfected user is a less costly user, and is not a risk for disease transmission to the broader community.

The overwhelming evidence is that such schemes reduce both drug- and sex-related risk behaviours (Cross *et al.*, 1998; Gibson *et al.*, 2001; Vlahov *et al.*, 2008; Wood *et al.*, 2007). There is also evidence that they reduce the HIV seroconversion rate among users, perhaps by as much as a third (Bastos & Strathdee, 2000; Gibson *et al.*, 2001; Pollack & Heimer, 2004; Vlahov & Junge, 1998). There is certainly no evidence to indicate that users inject more often, or are encouraged to use by the existence of such schemes. Needle provision appears to have been less successful in HCV prevention. Even in countries such as Australia, where it is commonly believed that needle provision averted an epidemic of HIV among IDU, HCV seroprevalence is high. This, in all probability, is due to the significantly higher infectivity of HCV discussed earlier. *Any* needle sharing episode will carry a high risk of HCV infection. Like all interventions, sterile needle provision is not a panacea. The evidence is, however, that it positively affects the health trajectories of many users, thus reducing subsequent direct and indirect costs to society.

9.2.4.2 *Overdose prevention*

We now move on to measures that directly relate to heroin users: the prevention of overdose and improving responses at such events. As we have seen, overdose is the major cause of premature death amongst heroin users, and non-fatal overdose is common and associated with a range of serious sequelae. The most obvious intervention is to educate heroin users about overdose risk. As we have seen, the most important fact to come out of overdose research in the last two decades is the prominent role of polydrug use. Educating heroin users on the risks of polydrug use may help reduce the frequency of overdose, as may education on the risk of overdosing after a period of abstinence. Indeed, it has been demonstrated that awareness of risk factors can be raised by means of such campaigns (McGregor *et al.*, 2001).

Improving heroin users' responses to overdoses may also reduce overdose morbidity and mortality, as we have seen that responses in these situations are typically very poor. Heroin users could be taught simple cardiopulmonary resuscitation skills so that they can keep overdose victims alive until help arrives. As pointed out to me by the director of a large treatment agency that provides such training, even if the person does not save another user, they may save their grandmother in an emergency. Users also need to be encouraged to call an ambulance immediately an overdose occurs, without risk of police intervention. It has been demonstrated that interventions of this type *can* improve the responses of heroin users, under circumstances where health and police have co-operated on emergency callouts (McGregor *et al.*, 2001).

While education is important, and has been implemented in many countries, a more controversial intervention is the provision of naloxone hydrochloride directly to heroin users (Darke & Hall, 2003; Lenton *et al.*, 2009; Lenton & Hargreaves, 2009; Strang *et al.*, 1999b, 2000). Naloxone hydrochloride is the narcotic antagonist used to reverse acute narcosis, and can be administered by intravenous, intramuscular, subcutaneous or intranasal routes. The major potential advantage of wider distribution is the increased chance of a comatose heroin user being quickly resuscitated. Importantly, naloxone has no pharmacological activity in the absence of opioids, and lacks any abuse potential. There is simply nothing else you can do with the drug, and it is difficult to imagine a black market emerging for an *anti*-intoxicant. Naloxone has been available as an over-the-counter drug in Italy since 1995, and also provided more directly to heroin users, but no formal evaluation has been conducted (Simini, 1998). Small-scale pilot distribution schemes have been conducted in Germany, Jersey and the USA in conjunction with broader resuscitation training (Dettmer *et al.*, 2001; Galea *et al.*, 2006; Seal *et al.*, 2005). All studies to date indicate that heroin users will take home supplies of naloxone if available, that they will use it appropriately, that they are able to reverse overdoses in emergencies and that adverse effects do not appear to be a problem.

Again, we must address the issue of whether it is morally acceptable to provide information and drugs to reduce overdose risk. Are we encouraging use? No, we are most certainly not. The only sure way to avoid a heroin overdose is not to use the drug. Given all we know of the long-term trajectories of heroin users, however, the risk of overdose is real, repeated and prolonged. Reducing rates of overdose-related morbidity and mortality may also be seen as a means to affect the trajectory, in this case by the avoidance of overdose death and/or other serious sequelae such as brain damage. Even if we ignore the moral imperative to provide succour to users, reducing overdose rates reduces the overall costs to society.

9.2.4.3 Medically supervised injecting centres

Finally, we will briefly examine the more contentious issue of medically supervised injecting centres. These are officially designated sites at which IDU can inject drugs without fear of arrest, where sterile injection equipment is provided and where medical assistance is available in case of overdose (Kral *et al.*, 2010). Essentially, these facilities may be viewed as being in the same family as needle and syringe programmes, except that supervised injection occurs on-site. Such facilities exist in a number of countries, including Switzerland (since 1986), Germany (1994), the Netherlands (1996), Australia (2001) and Canada (2003) (Fast *et al.*, 2008; Kimber *et al.*, 2003; Kimber & Dolan, 2007; Kral *et al.*, 2010). Evaluations of safe injecting rooms have reported their acceptability to IDU, reductions in needle sharing, reduced injecting and discarded equipment in surrounding streets, improved access to medical care and reductions in overdose rates (Fast *et al.*, 2008; Kerr *et al.*,

2005; Kral *et al.*, 2010; Wood *et al.*, 2006). It must be borne in mind that the majority of overdoses, fatal and non-fatal, occur in the home environment. As such, such facilities will be of greatest utility in locations where there is a substantial degree of street-based injecting. It will be recalled that street injecting carries a higher risk of overdose. The utility of such facilities also extends to the reduction of street-based injecting and public nuisance.

The controversy surrounding medically supervised injecting centres is similar to that of needle exchange. Apart from the 'not in my backyard' syndrome, there is concern that such centres aid and abet drug use, and injecting drug use in particular. Again, I would argue that such facilities should be seen in the light of altering trajectories. They are a recognition of the long-term mortality risk of the dependent user, and an attempt to intervene to keep the person alive. They also act as sterile injecting outlets, and as conduits to the health system. As with the other interventions seen in this section, they are means to reduce the costs of heroin use to the individual and society. They do *not* attempt to encourage or proselytise drug use. Rather, they are a recognition of the trajectories and risks of users.

Overall, we should view harm reduction measures as means to affect the use career. It is true that they are not means to curtail that career. They may, however, improve the prognosis for individual users, and reduce the costs to society associated with long-term, dependent heroin use.

9.3 Concluding remarks

We come now to the end of this journey through the life and times of a typical heroin user. As we have seen, this journey starts long before heroin use commences, and frequently involves an abusive and pathological childhood. The fact that substance use is engendered by such backgrounds should not surprise. Once the move into heroin occurs, the risk of a lifetime of dependence is extraordinarily high. Once dependence develops the person has, effectively, lost control over their drug use. We are thus not speaking of a 'life choice'. All we know of heroin use tells us that stepping out of the 'career' is extremely difficult, and would be for anyone unfortunate enough to develop heroin dependence. We must abandon the appealing notion of heroin use as a transitory phase of the young drug user, from which they will mature out. The maturation hypothesis is dead. The march of time and cohorts of heroin users killed it. While some users will have relatively short careers, the reality for most is long years of use, overdose, disease and treatment. The risk of death is very real from this most lethal of all drugs.

Given what we now know about the use career, we must tailor our expectations to meet this reality. An increasingly large component of the treatment of heroin users, for example, will be of the 'geriatric user', with all the clinical concerns involved in treating older patients, particularly in prescribing. We must, however, not lose hope. Interventions can, and do, provide enormous benefits to users and society. Even if we ignore the moral imperative to provide help to heroin users, interventions such as treatment and needle provision dramatically reduce the harms and costs to society.

Given all we have seen, early intervention and prevention amongst young people is crucial, particularly amongst the children of people with substance use problems. The trajectories of users are not inevitable. If we can prevent the start of the trajectory, we may change an entire life. For those who do commence use, while their careers may often be long, their trajectories *can* be changed for the better. As there is no one trajectory we, as a society and a treatment community, can make a difference.

Key points: Summary of conclusions: an inevitable life and death?

- Interventions need to be informed by knowledge of typical trajectories. Stable high-level use may occur over the course of decades.
- In any use career, significant turning points will occur, the two most salient being drug treatment enrolment and incarceration. These may be conceptualised as opportunities to deflect the trajectory towards reduced use and harm.
- Interventions to reduce harm fall into three broad categories: prevention, treatment and harm reduction.
- There is evidence to suggest that school-based drug education may have a significant effect in preventing or delaying drug use among young people.
- Long-term, stable retention is a consistent predictor of superior treatment outcome.
- The rationale for harm reduction measures lies in the chronicity of dependence, and its serious harms. Such measures include the provision of sterile injecting equipment, overdose prevention, and medically supervised injection centres.
- Harm reduction measures can be viewed as means to affect the user's trajectory, with resultant reduced cost to society.

References

Abdollahi, M. & Radfarl, M. (2003). A review of drug-induced oral reactions. *Journal of Contemporary Dental Practice, 4*, 10–31.

Abelson, J., Treloar, C., Crawford, J., Kippax, S., Van Beek, I. & Howard, J. (2006). Some characteristics of early-onset injection drug users prior to and at the time of their first injection. *Addiction, 101*, 548–555.

Aceijas, C., Stimson, G., Hickman, M. & Rhodes, T. (2004). Global overview of injecting drug use and HIV infection among injecting drug users. *AIDS, 18*, 2295–2303.

Aderjan, R., Hoemann, S., Schmitt, G. & Skopp, G. (1995). Morphine and morphine glucuronides in serum of heroin consumers and in heroin-related deaths determined by HPLC with native fluorescence detection. *Journal of Analytical Toxicology, 19*, 163–168.

Agrawal, A. & Lynskey, M. (2008). Are there genetic influences on addiction: evidence from family, adoption and twin studies. *Addiction, 103*, 1069–1081.

Agrawal, A., Neale, M. C., Prescott, C. A. & Kendler, K. S. (2004). Cannabis and other illicit drugs: comorbid use and abuse/dependence in males and females. *Behavior Genetics, 34*, 217–228.

Ahmadi, J. (2003). Methadone versus buprenorphine maintenance for the treatment of heroin-dependent outpatients. *Journal of Substance Abuse Treatment, 24*, 217–220.

Ahmadi, J., Arabi, H. & Mansouri, Y. (2003). Prevalence of substance use among offspring of opioid addicts. *Addictive Behaviors, 28*, 591–595.

Aitken, C., Kerger, M. & Crofts, N. (2000). Drivers who use illicit drugs: behaviour and perceived risks. *Drugs: Education, Prevention and Policy, 7*, 39–50.

Albery, I., Gossop, M., Strang, J. & Griffiths, P. (2000). Illicit drugs and driving: prevalence, beliefs and accident involvement among a cohort of current out-of-treatment drug users. *Drug and Alcohol Dependence, 58*, 197–204.

American Psychiatric Association. (2000). *Diagnostic and Statistical Manual of Mental Disorders (4th edn. Text Revision)*. Washington, DC: American Psychiatric Association.

Anglin, M. D., Brecht, M. L., Woodward, J. A. & Bonett, D. G. (1986). An empirical study of maturing out: conditional factors. *International Journal of the Addictions, 21*, 233–246.

Anglin, M. D., Speckart, G. R, Booth, M. W. & Ryan, T. M. (1989). Consequences and costs of shutting off methadone. *Addictive Behaviors, 14*, 307–326.

Anglin, M. D., Hser, Y. I. & Grella, C. E. (1997). Drug addiction and treatment careers among clients in the Drug Abuse Treatment Outcome Study (DATOS). *Psychology of Addictive Behaviors, 11*, 308–323.

Anthony, J. C., Warner, L. & Kessler, R. (1994). Comparative epidemiology of dependence on tobacco, alcohol, controlled substances, and inhalants: basic findings from the National Comorbidity Survey. *Experimental and Clinical Psychopharmacology, 2*, 244–268.

Antolini G., Pirani, M., Morandi, G. & Sorio, C. (2006). Gender differnce and mortality in a cohort of heroin users in the provinces of Modena and Ferrara, 1975–1999. *Epidemiologia e Preventione, 30*, 91–99.

Appleby, L., Cooper, J., Amos, T. & Faragher, B. (1999). Psychological autopsy study of suicides by people under 35. *British Journal of Psychiatry, 175*, 168–174.

Arriola, K. R. J., Louden, T., Doldren, M. A. & Fortenberry, R. M. (2005). A meta-analysis of the relationship of child sexual abuse to HIV risk behavior among women. *Child Abuse and Neglect, 29*, 725–746.

Athanasiadus, L. (1999). Drugs, alcohol and violence. *Current Opinion in Psychiatry, 12*, 281–286.

Auriacombe, M., Franque, P. & Tignol, J. (2001). Deaths attributable to methadone vs. buprenorphine in France. *Journal of American Medical Association, 285*, 45.

Australian Institute of Health and Welfare. (2008). *2007 National Household Survey: Detailed Findings*. Drug Statistics Series No. 16. Canberra: Australian Institute of Health and Welfare.

Azim, T., Chowdhury, E. I., Reza, M. *et al.* (2008). Prevalence of infections, HIV risk behaviors and factors associated with HIV infection among male injecting drug users attending a needle/syringe exchange program in Dhaka. *Bangladesh Substance Use and Misuse, 43*, 2124–2144.

Baca, C. T. & Grant, K. J. (2007). What heroin users tell us about overdose. *Journal of Addictive Diseases, 26*, 63–68.

Backmunda, M., Schuetzb, C., Meyera, K., Edlinc, B. R. & Reimer, J. (2009). The risk of emergency room treatment due to overdose in injection drug users. *Journal of Addictive Diseases, 28*, 68–73.

Bailey, R. C., Hser, Y. I. & Anglin, H. (1994). Influences affecting maintenance and cessation of narcotics addiction. *Journal of Drug Issues, 24*, 249–272.

Balakireva, O. & Grund, J. P. (2006). *Risk and Protective Factors in the Initiation of Injecting Drug Use*. Kiev: UNAIDS.

Ball, J. C. & Ross, A. (1991). *The Effectiveness of Methadone Maintenance Treatment: Patients, Programs, Services, and Outcome*. Vienna: Springer-Verlag.

Bammer, G. (2009). Treating heroin dependence with diamorphine (pharmaceutical heroin). In R. P. Mattick., R. Ali. & N. Lintzeris. (eds.) *Pharmacotherapies for the Treatment of Opioid Dependence: Efficacy, Cost-effectiveness, and Implementation Guidelines*, pp. 54–106. New York: Informa Healthcare.

Bargagli, A.M., Sperati, A., Davoli, F., Forastiere, F. & Perucci, C.A. (2001). Mortality among problem drug users in Rome: an 18-year follow-up study, 1980–1997. *Addiction*, *96*, 1455–1463.

Bargagli, A.M., Faggiano, F., Amato, L. *et al.* (2006). VEdeTTE, a longitudinal study on effectiveness of treatments for heroin addiction in Italy: study protocol and characteristics of study population. *Substance Use and Misuse*, *41*, 1861–1879.

Bargagli, A.M., Hickman, M., Davoli, M. *et al.* (2006). Drug-related mortality and its impact on adult mortality in eight European countries. *European Journal of Public Health*, *16*, 198–202.

Bartholomew, N.G., Courtney, K., Rowan-Szal, G.A. & Simpson, D.D. (2005). Sexual abuse history and treatment outcomes among women undergoing methadone treatment. *Journal of Substance Abuse Treatment*, *29*, 231–235.

Bartu, A., Freeman, N.C., Gawthorne, G.S., Allsop, S.J. & A.J. (2002). Characteristics, retention and readmissions of opioid-dependent clients treated with oral naltrexone. *Drug and Alcohol Review*, *21*, 335–340.

Bartu, A., Freeman, N.C., Gawthorne, G.S., Codde, J.P. & Holman, D.J. (2004). Mortality in a cohort of opiate and amphetamine users in Perth, Western Australia. *Addiction*, *99*, 63–60.

Bastos, F.I. & Strathdee, S. (2000). Evaluating effectivness of syringe exchange programmes: current issues and future prospects. *Social Science and Medicine*, *51*, 1771–1782.

Bauer, S.M., Loiple, R., Jagsch, R. *et al.* (2008). Mortality in opioid-maintained patients after release from an addiction clinic. *European Addiction Research*, *14*, 82–91.

Bell, J., Byron, G., Gibson, A. & Morris, A. (2004). A pilot study of buprenorphine–naloxone combination tablet (Suboxone®) in treatment of opioid dependence. *Drug and Alcohol Review*, *23*, 311–317. http://onlinelibrary.wiley.com/doi/ 10.1080/09595230412331289473/abstract – fn1

Bell, J., Shanahan, M., Mutch, C. *et al.* (2007). A randomized trial of effectiveness and cost-effectiveness of observed versus unobserved administration of bupre-norphine–naloxone for heroin dependence. *Addiction*, *102*, 1899–1907.

Bennett, G. & Higgins, D. (1999). Accidental overdose among injecting drug users in Dorset, UK. *Addiction*, *94*, 1179–1190.

Bertelote, J.M. & Fleischmann, A. (2002). A global perspective in the epidemiology of suicide. *Suicidologi*, *7*, 6–8.

Best, D., Gossop, M., Lehmann, P., Harris, J. & Strang, J. (1999). The relationship between overdose and alcohol consumption among methadone maintenance patients. *Journal of Substance Use*, *4*, 41–44.

Best, D., Gossop, M., Man, L., Stillwell, G., Coomber, R. & Strang, J. (2002). Peer overdose resuscitation: multiple intervention strategies and time to response by drug users who witness overdose. *Drug and Alcohol Review*, *21*, 269–274.

Beynon, C. M., Roe, B., Duffy, P. & Pickering, L. (2009). Self reported health status, and health service contact, of illicit drug users aged 50 and over: a qualitative interview study in Merseyside, United Kingdom. *BMC Geriatrics*, *9*, 45.

Bird, S. M. (2010). Over 1200 drugs-related deaths and 190,000 opiate-users-years of follow-up: relative risks by sex and age group. *Addiction Research and Theory*, *18*, 194–207.

Bjornaas, M. A., Bekken, A. S., Ojlert, A. *et al.* (2008). A 20-year prospective study of mortality and causes of death among hospitalized opioid addicts in Oslo. *BMC Psychiatry*, *8*, 1–8.

Bobashev, G. V. & Anthony, J. C. (1998). Clusters of marijuana use in the United States. *American Journal of Epidemiology*, *148*, 1168–1174.

Boeri, M. W., Sterk, C. E. & Eklifson, K. W. (2008). Reconceptualizing early and late onset: a life course analysis of older heroin users. *The Gerontologist*, *48*, 637–645.

Boles, S. M. & Miotto, K. (2003). Substance abuse and violence: a review of the literature. *Aggression and Violent Behaviour*, *8*, 155–174.

Borges, G., Walters, E. E. & Kessler, R. C. (2000). Associations of substance use, abuse, and dependence with subsequent suicidal behaviour. *American Journal of Epidemiology*, *151*, 781–789.

Botvin, G. & Griffin K. W. (2007). School-based programs to prevent alcohol, tobacco and other drug use. *International Review of Psychiatry*, *19*, 607–15.

Boyd, J., Randell, T., Luurila, H. & Kuisma, M. (2003). Serious overdoses involving buprenorphine in Helsinki. *Acta Anaestiologica Scandinavia*, *47*, 1031–1033.

Bradley, R. H. & Corwyn, R. F. (2002). Socioeconomic status and child development. *Annual Review of Psychology*, *53*, 371–399.

Brådvik, L., Hulenvik, P., Frank, A., Medvedeo, A. & Berglund, M. (2007). Self-reported and observed heroin overdoses in Malmoe. *Journal of Substance Use*, *12*, 119–126.

Braitstein, P., Lia, K., Tyndall, M. *et al.* (2003). Sexual violence among a cohort of injection drug users. *Social Science & Medicine*, *57*, 561–569.

Branstetter, S. A., Bower, E. H., Kamien, J. & Amass, L. (2008). A history of sexual, emotional, or physical abuse predicts adjustment during opioid maintenance treatment. *Journal of Substance Abuse Treatment*, *34*, 208–214.

Breslau, N. N., Scott, P. & Kessler, R. C. (2004). Psychiatric disorders and stages of smoking. *Biological Psychiatry*, *55*, 69–76.

Brienza, R. S., Stein, M. D., Chen, M. H. *et al.* (2000). Depression among needle exchange and methadone maintenance clients. *Journal of Substance Abuse Treatment*, *18*, 331–337.

Britton, P. C., Wines, J. D. & Conner, K. R. (2010). Non-fatal overdose in the 12 months following treatment for substance use disorders. *Drug and Alchol Dependence*, *107*, 51–55.

Broome, K. M., Joe, G. W. & Simpson, D. D. (1999). Patient and program attributes related to treatment process indicators in DATOS. *Drug and Alcohol Dependence*, *57*, 127–135.

Brooner, R. K., Greenfield, L., Schmidt, C. W. & Bigelow, G. E. (1993). Antisocial personality disorder and HIV infection in drug abusers. *American Journal of Psychiatry*, *150*, 53–58.

Brugal, M. T., Barrio, G., de la Fuente, L. Regidor, E., Royuela, L. & Suelves, J. M. (2002). Factors associated with non-fatal heroin overdose: assessing the effect of frequency and route of heroin administration. *Addiction*, *97*, 319–327.

Brugal, M. T., Domingo-Salvany, A., Puig, R. *et al.* (2005). Evaluating the impact of methadone maintenance programmes on mortality due to overdose and AIDS in a cohort of heroin users in Spain. *Addiction*, *100*, 981–989.

Bryant, W. K., Galea, S., Tracy, M., Piper, T. M., Tardiff, K. J. & Vlahov, D. (2003). Overdose deaths attributed to methadone and heroin in New York City, 1990–1998. *Addiction*, *99*, 846–854.

Budd, J., Copeland, L., Elton, R. & Robertson, R. (2002). Hepatitis C infection in a cohort of injecting drug users: past and present risk factors and the implications for educational and clinical management. *European Journal of General Practice*, *8*, 95–100.

Bull, S. S., Piper, P. & Rietmeijer, C. (2002). Men who have sex with men and also inject drugs – profiles of risk related to the synergy of sex and drug injection behaviors. *Journal of Homosexuality*, *42*, 31–51.

Burns, J. M., Martyres, R. F., Clode, D. & Boldero, J. M. (2004). Overdose in young people using heroin: associations with mental health, prescription drug use and personal circumstances. *Medical Journal of Australia*, *181*, S25–S28.

Burns, L., Conroy, E. & Mattick, R. P. (2010). Infant mortality among women on a methadone program during pregnancy. *Drug and Alcohol Review*, *29*, 551–556.

Buster, M. C. A., Rook, L., van Brussel, H. A., van Ree, J. & van den Brink, W. (2002). Chasing the dragon related to impaired lung function among heroin users. *Drug and Alcohol Dependence*, *68*, 221–228.

Cacciola, J. S., Alterman, A. I., Rutherford, M. J., McKay, J. R. & Mulvaney, F. D. (2001). The relationship of psychiatric comorbidity to treatment outcomes in methadone maintained patients. *Drug and Alcohol Dependence*, *61*, 271–280.

Calabria, B., Degenhardt, L., Briegleb, C. *et al.* (2010). Systematic review of prospective studies investigating 'remission' from amphetamine, cannabis, cocaine or opioid dependence. *Addictive Behaviors*, *35*, 741–749.

Carpenter, M. J., Chutuape, M. A. & Stitzer, M. L. (1998). Heroin snorters versus injectors: comparison on drug use and treatment outcome in age-matched samples. *Drug and Alcohol Dependence*, *53*, 11–15.

Carpentier, P. J., Krabbe, P. F. M., van Gogh, M. T., Knapen, L. J. M., Buitelaar, J. K. & de Jong, C. A. J. (2009). Psychiatric comorbidity reduces quality of life in chronic methadone maintained patients. *The American Journal on Addictions*, *18*, 470–480.

Caputo, F., Addolorato, G., Domenicali, M. *et al.* (2002). Short-term methadone administration reduces alcohol consumption in non-alcoholic heroin addicts. *Alcohol and Alcoholism*, *37*, 164–168. http://alcalc.oxfordjournals.org/content/37/2/164.full – aff-5

Carise, D., Dugosh, K. L., McLellan, A. T., Camilleri, A., Woody, G. E. & Lynch, K. G. (2007). Prescription oxycontin abuse among patients entering addiction treatment. *American Journal of Psychiatry*, *164*, 1750–1756.

Cecile, J.S, Alderman, A.I, Rutherford, M.J, McKay, J. R. & Mulvane, F. D. (2001). The relationship of psychiatric comorbidity to treatment outcomes in methadone maintained patients. *Drug Alcohol Dependence*, *61*, 271–280.

Chaisson, R. E., Bacchetti, P., Osmond, D., Brodie, B., Sande, M. A. & Moss, A. R. (1989). Cocaine use and HIV infection in intravenous drug users in San Francisco. *Journal of the American Medical Association*, *261*, 561–565.

Chatham, L. R., Knight, K., Joe, G. W. & Simpson, D. D. (1995). Suicidality in a sample of methadone maintenance patients. *American Journal of Drug and Alcohol Abuse*, *21*, 345–361.

Chen, K. & Kandel, D. B. (1995). The natural history of drug use from adolescence to the mid-thirties in a general population sample. *American Journal of Public Health*, *85*, 41–47.

Chen, V. C., Lin, T. Y., Lee, C. T. *et al.* (2010). Suicide attempts prior to starting methadone maintenance treatment in Taiwan. *Drug and Alcohol Dependence* *109*, 139–143.

Chiang, S., Chua, Chen, S. J., Sun, H. J., Chan, H. Y. & Chen, W. J. (2006). Heroin use among youths incarcerated for illicit drug use: psychosocial environment, substance use history, psychiatric comorbidity, and route of administration. *The American Journal on Addictions*, *15*, 233–241.

Cicchetti, D. & Rogosch, F. A. (1999). Psychopathology as risk for adolescent substance use disorders: a developmental psychopathology perspective. *Journal of Clinical Child Psychology*, *28*, 355–365.

Cicero, T., Inciardi, J. & Muñoz, A. (2005). Trends in abuse of oxycontin® and other opioid analgesics in the United States: 2002–2004. *Journal of Pain*, *6*, 662–672.

City of Vancouver. (2008). Methadone becoming a nursing-home drug. *Four Pillars News*. City of Vancouver For Pillars Coalition Newsletter. September, 2008.

Clark, D. B., Thatcher, D. L. & Tapert, S. F. (2008). Alcohol, psychological dysregulation, and adolescent brain development. *Alcoholism: Clinical Experimental Research*, *32*, 378–385.

Clark, H. W., Masson, C. L., Deluchi, K. L., Hall, S. M. & Sees, K. L. (2001). Violent traumatic events and drug abuse severity. *Journal of Substance Abuse Treatment*, *20*, 121–127.

Clarke, T. K., Krause, K., Li, T. & Schumann, G. (2009). An association of prodynorphin polymorphisms and opioid dependence in females in a Chinese population. *Biology*, *14*, 366–370.

Clausen, T., Anchersen, K. & Waal, H. (2008). Mortality prior to, during and after opioid maintenance treatment (OMT): a national prospective cross-registry study. *Drug and Alcohol Dependence, 94*, 151–157.

Clausen, T., Waal, H, Thoresen, M. & Gossop, M. (2009). Mortality among opiate users: opioid maintenance therapy, age and causes of death. *Addiction, 104*, 1356–1362.

Coffin, P. O., Tracy, M., Bucciarelli, A., Ompad, D., Vlahov, D. & Galea, S. (2007). Identifying injecting drug users at risk of non-fatal overdose. *Academic Emergency Medicine, 14*, 616–623.

Collins, D., Lapsley, H. & Marks, R. (2007). *The Three Billion $ Question for Australian Business.* Sydney: Australian Drug Law Reform Foundation.

Conroy, E., Degenhardt, L., Mattick, R. P. & Nelson, E. C. (2009). Child maltreatment as a risk factor for opioid dependence: comparison of family characteristics and type and severity of child maltreatment with a matched control group. *Child Abuse and Neglect, 33*, 343–352.

Cook, S., Moeschler, O., Michaud, K. & Yersin, B. (1998). Acute opiate overdose: characteristics of 190 consecutive cases. *Addiction, 93*, 1559–1569.

Coomber, R. (1999). The cutting of heroin in the United States in the 1990s. *Journal of Drug Issues, 29*, 17–36.

Cooncool, B., Smith, H. & Stimmel, B. (1979). Mortality rates of persons entering methadone maintenance: a seven-year study. *American Journal of Drug and Alcohol Abuse, 6*, 345–353.

Costello, E., Erkanli, A., Federman, E. & Angold, A. (1999). Development of psychiatric comorbidity with substance abuse in adolescents: effects of timing and sex. *Journal of Clinical Child Psychology, 28*, 298–311.

Cottler, L. B., Compson, W. M., Mager, D., Spitznagel, E. L. & Janca, A. (1992). Posttraumatic stress disorder among substance abusers from the general population. *American Journal of Psychiatry, 149*, 664–670.

Courtwright, D., Joseph, H. & Des Jarlais, D. (1989). *Addicts Who Survived: An Oral History of Narcotic Addiction in America 1923–1965.* Knoxville: University of Tennessee.

Coviello, D. M., Alterman, A. I., Cacciola, J. S., Rutherford, M. J. & Zanis, D. A. (2004). The role of family history in addiction severity and treatment response. *Journal of Substance Abuse Treatment, 26*, 1–11.

Cox, G. & Comiskey, C. M. (2007). Baseline characteristics of patients attending treatment for opiate use in Ireland. *Drugs: Education, Prevention and Policy, 14*, 217–230.

Crofts, N., Louie, R., Rosenthal, D. & Jolley, D. (1996). The first hit: circumstances surrounding initiation into injecting. *Addiction, 91*, 1187–1196.

Crofts, N., Aitken, C. & Kaldor, J. (1999). The force of numbers: why hepatitis C is spreading among Australian injecting drug users while HIV is not. *Medical Journal of Australia, 170*, 220–221.

Cross, J.C., Saunders, C. & Bartelli, D. (1998). The effectiveness of educational and needle exchange programs: a meta-analysis of HIV prevention strategies for injecting drug users. *Quality and Quantity, 32*, 165–180.

Cuijpers P. (2002). Effective ingredients of school-based drug prevention programs. A systematic review. *Addictive Behaviors, 27*, 1009–23.

Cumming, S., Covic, T. & Murrell, E. (2006). Deliberate self-harm: have we scratched the surface? *Behaviour Change, 23*, 186–99.

Curran, C., Byrappa, N. & McBride, A. (2004). Stimulant psychosis: systematic review. *British Journal of Psychiatry, 185*, 196–204.

Cynan, J., Trunsky, M. & Cobridge, T. (2000). Inhaled heroin-induced status asthmaticus: five cases and a review of the literature. *Chest, 117*, 272–275.

Daniel, A. Z., Hickman, M., McLeod, J *et al.* (2009) Is socioeconomic status in early life associated with drug use? A systematic review of the evidence. *Drug and Alcohol Review, 28*, 142–153.

Darke, S. (2010). The toxicology of homicide offenders and victims: a review. *Drug and Alcohol Review, 29*, 202–215.

Darke, S. & Duflou, J. (2008). Toxicology and circumstances of death of homicide victims in New South Wales, Australia 1996–2005. *Journal of Forensic Sciences, 53*, 447–451.

Darke, S. & Hall, W. (2003). Heroin overdose: research and evidence-based intervention. *Journal of Urban Health, 80*, 189–200.

Darke, S. & Ross, J. (1997). Polydrug dependence and psychiatric comorbidity among heroin injectors. *Drug and Alcohol Dependence, 48*, 135–141.

Darke, S & Ross, J. (2000). Fatal heroin overdoses resulting from non-injecting routes of administration, NSW, Australia, 1992–1996. *Addiction, 95*, 596–599.

Darke, S. & Ross, J. (2001). The relationship between suicide and overdose among methadone maintenance patients in Sydney, Australia. *Addiction, 96*, 1443–1453.

Darke, S. & Ross, J. (2002). Suicide among heroin users: rates, risk factors and methods. *Addiction, 97*, 1383–1394.

Darke, S., Ross, J. & Hall, W. (1996a). Prevalence and correlates of the injection of methadone syrup in Sydney, Australia. *Drug and Alcohol Dependence, 43*, 191–198.

Darke, S., Ross, J. & Hall, W. (1996b). Overdose among heroin users in Sydney, Australia I. Prevalence and correlates of non-fatal overdose. *Addiction, 91*, 405–411.

Darke, S., Ross, J. & Hall, W. (1996c). Overdose among heroin users in Sydney, Australia II. Responses to overdose. *Addiction, 91*, 413–417.

Darke, S., Sunjic, S., Zador, D. & Prolov, T. (1997). A comparison of blood toxicology of heroin-related deaths and current heroin users in Sydney, Australia. *Drug and Alcohol Dependence, 47*, 45–53.

Darke, S., Kaye, S. & Finlay-Jones, R. (1998). Antisocial personality disorder, psychopathy and injecting drug use. *Drug and Alcohol Dependence, 52*, 63–69.

Darke, S., Hall, W., Weatherburn, D. & Lind, B. (1999a). Fluctuations in heroin purity and the incidence of fatal heroin overdose. *Drug and Alcohol Dependence*, *54*, 155–161.

Darke, S., Kaye, S. & Ross, J. (1999b). Transitions between the injection of heroin and amphetamines. *Addiction*, *94*, 1795–1803.

Darke, S., Ross, J., Zador, D. & Sunjic, S. (2000). Heroin-related deaths in New South Wales, Australia, 1992–1996. *Drug and Alcohol Dependence*, *60*, 141–150.

Darke, S., Kaye, S. & Ross, J. (2001a). Geographical injecting locations among injecting drug users in Sydney, Australia. *Addiction*, *96*, 241–246.

Darke, S., Ross, J. & Kaye, S. (2001b). Physical injecting sites among injecting drug users in Sydney, Australia. *Drug and Alcohol Dependence*, *62*, 77–82.

Darke, S., Hall, W., Kaye, S., Ross, J. & Duflou, J. (2002a). Hair morphine concentrations of fatal heroin overdose cases and living heroin users. *Addiction*, *97*, 977–984.

Darke, S., Topp, L. & Ross, J. (2002b). The injection of methadone and benzodiazepines among Sydney IDU 1996–2000: 5 year monitoring of trends from the Illicit Drug Reporting System (IDRS). *Drug and Alcohol Review*, *21*, 35–40.

Darke, S., Kelly, E. & Ross, J. (2003a). Drug use and driving among injecting drug users in Sydney, Australia: prevalence, risk factors and risk perceptions. *Addiction*, *99*, 175–185.

Darke, S., Mattick, R. & Degenhardt, L. (2003b). The ratio of non-fatal to fatal overdose. *Addiction*, *98*, 1169–1170.

Darke, S., Ross, J. & Lynskey, M. (2003c). The relationship of conduct disorder to attempted suicide and drug use history among methadone maintenance patients. *Drug and Alcohol Review*, *22*, 21–25.

Darke, S., Hetherington, K., Ross, J., Lynskey, M. & Teesson, M. (2004a). Non-injecting routes of administration among entrants to three treatment modalities for heroin dependence. *Drug and Alcohol Review*, *23*, 177–183.

Darke, S., Ross, J., Lynskey, M. & Teesson, M. (2004b). Attempted suicide among entrants to three treatment modalities for heroin dependence in the Australian Treatment Outcome Study (ATOS): prevalence and risk factors. *Drug and Alcohol Dependence*, *73*, 1–10.

Darke, S., Williamson, A., Ross, J., Teesson, M. & Lynskey, M. (2004c). Borderline personality disorder, antisocial personality disorder and risk-taking among heroin users: findings from the Australian Treatment Outcome Study (ATOS). *Drug and Alcohol Dependence*, *74*, 77–83.

Darke, S., Kaye, S. & Duflou, J. (2005a). Cocaine-related fatalities in New South Wales, Australia 1993–2002. *Drug Alcohol Dependence*, *77*, 107–114.

Darke, S., Ross, J. & Teesson, M. (2005b). Twelve month outcomes for heroin dependence treatments: does route of administration matter? *Drug and Alcohol Review*, *24*, 165–171.

Darke, S., Ross, J., Teesson, M., Ali, R., Cooke, R., Ritter, A. & Lynskey, M. (2005c). Factors associated with 12 months continuous heroin abstinence: findings from the Australian Treatment Outcome Study (ATOS). *Journal of Substance Abuse Treatment, 28*, 255–263.

Darke, S., Ross, J., Williamson, A. & Teesson, M. (2005d). The impact of Borderline Personality Disorder on 12 month outcomes for the treatment of heroin dependence. *Addiction, 100*, 1121–1130.

Darke, S., Kaye, S. & Duflou, J. (2006a). Systemic disease among cases of fatal opioid toxicity. *Addiction, 101*, 1299–1305.

Darke, S., Williamson, A., Ross, J. & Teesson, M. (2006b). Residential rehabilitation for the treatment of heroin dependence: sustained heroin abstinence and drug-related problems two years after treatment entrance. *Addictive Disorders and Their Treatment, 5*, 9–18.

Darke, S., Williamson, A., Ross, J. & Teesson, M. (2006c). Reductions in heroin use are not associated with increases in other drug use: two year findings from the Australian Treatment Outcome Study. *Drug and Alcohol Dependence, 84*, 201–205.

Darke, S., Degenhardt, L. & Mattick, R. (2007a). *Mortality Amongst Illicit Drug Users: Epidemiology, Causes and Intervention*. Cambridge: Cambridge University Press.

Darke, S., Havard, A., Ross, J., Williamson, A., Mills, K. L. & Teesson, M. (2007b). Changes in the use of medical services and prescription drugs amongst heroin users over two years. *Drug and Alcohol Review, 26*, 153–159.

Darke, S., Ross, J., Mills, K. L., Williamson, A., Havard, A. & Teesson, M. (2007c). Borderline Personality Disorder and persistently elevated levels of risk in 36 month outcomes. *Addiction, 102*, 1140–1146.

Darke, S., Ross, J., Mills, K. L., Williamson, A., Havard, A. & Teesson, M. (2007d). Patterns of sustained heroin abstinence amongst long-term, dependent heroin users: 36 months findings from the Australian Treatment Outcome Study (ATOS). *Addictive Behaviors, 32*, 1897–1906.

Darke, S., Ross, J., Williamson, A., Mills, K. L., Havard, A. & Teesson, M. (2007e). Patterns of non-fatal heroin overdose over a three year period: findings from the Australian Treatment Outcome Study. *Journal of Urban Health, 84*, 283–291.

Darke, S., Ross, J., Williamson, A., Mills, K. L., Havard, A. & Teesson, M. (2007f). Patterns and correlates of attempted suicide by heroin users over a three year period: findings from the Australian Treatment Outcome Study. *Drug and Alcohol Dependence, 87*, 146–152.

Darke, S., Kaye, S., McKetin, R. & Duflou, J. (2008a). The major physical and psychological harms of methamphetamine use. *Drug and Alcohol Review, 27*, 253–262.

Darke, S., Ross, J., Mills, K. L., Williamson, A., Havard, A. & Teesson, M. (2008b). Injecting and non-injecting heroin administration: transitions and treatment outcomes across 36 months. *Journal of Drug Issues, 38*, 543–558.

Darke, S., Duflou, J. & Torok, M. (2009a). Toxicology and circumstances of completed suicide by means other than overdose. *Journal of Forensic Sciences, 54*, 490–494.

Darke, S., Mills, K. L., Ross, J., Teesson, M., Williamson, A. & Havard, A. (2009b). Patterns of major depression and drug-related problems amongst heroin users across 36 months. *Psychiatric Research, 166*, 7–14.

Darke, S., Mills, K. L., Ross, J., Williamson, A., Havard, A. & Teesson, M. (2009c). The ageing heroin user: career length, clinical profile and outcomes across 36 months. *Drug and Alcohol Review, 28*, 243–249.

Darke, S., Duflou, J. & Torok, M. (2010a). The comparative toxicology and major organ pathology of fatal methadone and heroin toxicity cases. *Drug and Alcohol Dependence, 106*, 1–6.

Darke, S., Duflou, J. & Torok, M. (2010b). Comparative toxicology of intentional and accidental heroin overdose. *Journal of Forensic Sciences, 55*, 1015–1018.

Darke, S., Ross, J., Mills, K., Teesson, M., Williamson, A. & Havard, A. (2010c). Benzodiazepine use amongst heroin users: baseline use, current use and clinical outcome. *Drug and Alcohol Review, 29*, 250–255.

Darke, S., Torok, M., Kaye, S., & Ross, J. (2010d). Attempted suicide, self-harm and violent victimisation amongst regular illicit drug users. *Suicide and Life-Threatening Behavior, 40*, 587–596.

Darke, S., Torok, M., Kaye, S., Ross, J. & McKetin, R. (2010e). Comparative rates of violent crime amongst regular methamphetamine and opioid users: offending and victimisation. *Addiction, 105*, 916–919.

Darke, S., Duflou, J. & Torok, M. (2011). Toxicology and characteristics of fatal oxycodone toxicity cases in New South Wales, Australia 1999–2008. *Journal of Forensic Sciences, 54*, 490–494.

Darke, S., Mills, K. L., Ross, J. & Teesson, M. (in press b). Rates and correlates of mortality amongst heroin users: findings from the Australian Treatment Outcome Study (ATOS), 2001–2009. *Drug and Alcohol Dependence*.

Davidson, P. J., McLean, R. L., Kral, A. H., Gleghorn, A. A., Edlin, B. R. & Moss, A. R. (2003). Fatal heroin-related overdose in San Francisco, 1997–2000: a case for targeted intervention. *Journal of Urban Health: Bulletin of the New York Academy of Medicine, 80*, 261–273.

Davoli, M., Perucci, C. A., Rapiti, E. *et al.* (1997). A persistent rise in mortality among injection drug users in Rome, 1980 through 1992. *American Journal of Public Health, 87*, 851–853.

Davoli, M., Bargagli, A. M., Perucci, C. A. *et al.* (2007). Risk of fatal overdose during and after specialist drug treatment: the VEdeTTE study, a national multisite prospective cohort study. *Addiction, 102*, 1954–1959.

Day, C., Degenhardt, L., Gilmour, S. & Hall, W. (2004). Effects of a reduction in heroin supply on injecting drug use: analysis of data from needle and syringe programmes. *British Medical Journal, 329*, 428–429.

Dean, A., Bell, J., Christie, M. J. & Mattick, R. P. (2004). Depressive symptoms during buprenorphine vs. methadone maintenance: findings from a randomised, controlled trial in opioid dependence. *European Psychiatry, 19*, 510–513.

Degenhardt, L. & Hall, W. (2002). Cannabis and psychosis. *Current Psychiatry Reports*, *4*, 191–196.

Degenhardt, L., Lynskey, M. & Hall, W. (2000). Cohort trends in the age of initiation of drug use in Australia. *Australian and New Zealand Journal of Public Health*, *24*, 421–426.

Degenhardt, L., Hall, W. & Lynskey, M. (2003). Testing hypotheses about the relationship between cannabis use and psychosis. *Drug and Alcohol Dependence*, *71*, 37–48.

Degenhardt, L., Hall, W., Warner-Smith, M. & Lynskey, M. (2004). Illicit drug use. In M. Ezzati, A. Lopez, A. Rodgers, & C. J. L. Murray. (eds.) *Comparative Quantification of Health Risks. Global and Regional Burden of Disease Attributable to Selected Major Risk Factors*. Vol **1**, pp. 1111–1175. Geneva: World Health Organization.

Degenhardt, L., Tennant, C., Gilmour, S. *et al.* (2007). The temporal dynamics of relationships between cannabis, psychosis and depression among young adults with psychotic disorders: findings from a 10-month prospective study. *Psychological Medicine*, *37*, 927–934.

Degenhardt, L., Kinner, S., Roxburgh, A. *et al.* (2008). Drug use and risk among regular injecting drug users in Australia: does age make a difference? *Drug and Alcohol Review*, *27*, 357–360.

Degenhardt, L., Chiu, W. T., Conway, K. *et al.* (2009a). Does the 'gateway' matter? Associations between the order of drug use initiation and the development of drug dependence in the National Comorbidity Study Replication. *Psychological Medicine*, *39*, 157–167.

Degenhardt, L., Randall, D., Hall, W., Law, M., Butler, T. & Burns, L. (2009b). Mortality among clients of a state-wide opioid pharmacotherapy program over 20 years: risk factors and lives saved. *Drug and Alcohol Dependence*, *105*, 9–15.

Degenhardt, L., Dierkerb, L., Chiu, W. T. *et al.* (2010). Evaluating the drug use 'gateway' theory using cross-national data: consistency and associations of the order of initiation of drug use among participants in the WHO World Mental Health Surveys. *Drug and Alchol Dependence*, *108*, 84–97.

Degenhardt, L., Bucello, C., Mathers, B. *et al.* (2011). Mortality among regular or dependent users of heroin and other opioids: a systematic review and meta-analysis of cohort studies. *Addiction*, *106*, 32–51.

de la Fuente, L., Saavedra, P., Barrio, G., Royuela, L. & Vicente, J. (1996). Temporal geographic variations in the characteristics of heroin seized in Spain and their relation with the route of administration. *Drug and Alcohol Dependence*, *40*, 185–194.

DeLeon, G., Melnick, G. & Cleland, C. (2008). Client matching: a severity-treatment intensity paradigm. *Journal of Addictive Disorders*, *27*, 99–111.

De los Cobos, J. P. (2007). Association of CYP2D6 ultrarapid metabolizer genotype with deficient patient satisfaction regarding methadone maintenance treatment. *Drug and Alcohol Dependence*, *89*, 190–194.

DeMaria, P. A., Sterling, R. & Weinstein, S. P. (2000). The effect of stimulant and sedative use on treatment outcome of patients admitted to methadone maintenance treatment. *American Journal of Addiction, 9,* 145–153.

Desmond, D. P., Maddux, J. F. & Trevino, A. (1978). Street heroin potency and deaths from overdose in San Antonio. *American Journal of Drug and Alcohol Abuse, 5,* 39–49.

Dettmer, K., Saunders, B. & Strang, J. (2001). Take home naloxone and the prevention of deaths from opiate overdose: two pilot schemes. *British Medical Journal, 322,* 895–896.

Deykin, E. Y. & Buka, S. L. (1994). Suicidal ideation and attempts among chemically dependent adolescents. *American Journal of Public Health, 84,* 634–639.

Dhossche, D. M., Rich, C. L., Ghani, S. O. & Isacson, G. (2001). Patterns of psychoactive substance detection from routine toxicology of suicides in Mobile, Alabama, between 1990 and 1998. *Journal of Affective Disorders, 64,* 167–174.

Diekstra, R. F. W. (1996). The epidemiology of suicide and parasuicide. *Archives of Suicide Research, 2,* 1–29.

Digiusto, E., Shakeshaft, A., Ritter, A., O'Brien, S., Mattick, R. P. & the-NEPOD-Research-Group (2004). Serious adverse events in the Australian National Evaluation of Pharmacotherapies for Opioid Dependence (NEPOD). *Addiction, 99,* 450–460.

Dinwiddie, S. H., Cottler, L., Compton, W. & Abdallah, A. B. (1996). Psychopathology and HIV risk behaviours among injection drug users in and out of treatment. *Drug and Alcohol Dependence, 43,* 1–11.

Doherty, M. C., Garfein, R. S., Monterroso, E., Brown, D. & Vlahov, D. (2000). Correlates of HIV infection among young adult short-term injection drug users. *AIDS, 14,* 717–726.

Dolan, K., Shearer, J., MacDonald, M., Mattick, R. P., Hall, W. & Wodak, A. D. (2003). A randomised controlled trial of methadone maintenance treatment versus wait list control in an Australian prison system. *Drug and Alcohol Dependence, 72,* 59–65.

Dolan, K. A., Shearer, J., White, B., Zhou, J., Kaldor, J. & Wodak, A. D. (2005). Four-year follow-up of imprisoned male heroin users and methadone treatment: mortality, re-incarceration and hepatitis C infection. *Addiction, 100,* 820–828.

Dole, V. P. & Nyswander, M. E. (1965). Medical treatment for diacetylmorphine (heroin) addiction. A clinical trial with methadone hydrochloride. *Journal of the American Medical Association, 193,* 646–650.

Dole, V. P., Nyswander, M. E. & Kreek, M. J. (1966). Narcotic blockade. *Archives of Internal Medicine, 118,* 304–309.

Drakenberg, K., Nikoshkov, A., Horvath, M. C. *et al.* (2006). mu opioid receptor A118G polymorphism in association with striatal opioid neuropeptide gene expression in heroin abusers. *Proceedings of the National Academy of Sciences, 103,* 7883–7888.

Dube, S. R., Anda, R. F., Whitfield, C. L. *et al.* (2005). Long-term consequences of childhood sexual abuse by gender of victim. *American Journal of Preventive Medicine*, *28*, 430–438.

Ellgren, M., Spano, S. M. & Hurd, Y. L. (2007). Adolescent cannabis exposure alters opiate intake and opioid limbic neuronal populations in adult rats. *Neuropsychopharmacology*, *32*, 607–615.

European Monitoring Centre for Drugs and Drug Addiction (2010). *Annual Report on the State of the Drugs Problem in Europe*. Lisbon: EMCDDA.

Evren, C. & Evren, B. (2005). Self-mutilation in substance-dependent patients and relationship with childhood abuse and neglect, alexithymia and temperament and character dimensions of personality. *Drug and Alcohol Dependence*, *80*, 15–22.

Fairbank, J. A., Dunteman, G. H. & Condelli, W. S. (1993). Do methadone patients substitute other drugs for heroin? Predicting substance use at 1-year follow-up. *American Journal of Drug and Alcohol Abuse*, *19*, 465–474.

Fajemirokun-Odudeyi, O., Sinha, C., Tutty, S. *et al.* (2006). Pregnancy outcome in women who use opiates. *European Journal of Obstetrics and Gynecology and Reproductive Biology*, *126*, 170–175.

Farrell, M. & Marsden, J. (2008). Acute risk of drug-related death among newly released prisoners in England and Wales. *Addiction*, *103*, 251–255.

Farrell, M., Boys, A., Bebbington, P. *et al.* (2002). Psychosis and drug dependence: results from a national survey of prisoners. *British Journal of Psychiatry*, *181*, 393–398.

Farrugia, P., Mills, K. L., Barrett, E. *et al.* (in press). Childhood trauma among individuals with co-morbid substance use and post traumatic stress disorder. *Mental Health & Substance Use: Dual Diagnosis*.

Fast, D. Small, W. Wood, E. & Kerr, T. (2008). The perspectives of injection drug users regarding safer injecting education delivered through a supervised injecting facility. *Harm Reduction Journal*, *5*, 32.

Fergus, S. & Zimmerman, M. A. (2005). Adolescent resilience: a framework for understanding healthy development in the face of risk. *Annual Review of Public Health*, *26*, 399–419.

Fergusson, D. M. & Horwood, L. J. (1997). Early onset cannabis use and psychosocial adjustment in young adults. *Addiction*, *92*, 279–296.

Fergusson, D. M. & Horwood, L. J. (2000). Does cannabis use encourage other forms of illicit drug use? *Addiction*, *95*, 505–520.

Fergusson, D. M. & Lynskey, M. T. (1995). Childhood circumstances, adolescent adjustment, and suicide attempts in a New Zealand Birth Cohort. *Journal of the American Academy of Child and Adolescent Psychiatry*, *34*, 612–622.

Fergusson, D. M. & Lynskey, M. T. (1997). Physical punishment/maltreatment during childhood and adjustment in young adulthood. *Child Abuse and Neglect*, *21*, 617–630.

Fergusson, D. M., Lynskey, M. T. & Horwood, L. J. (1993). Conduct problems and attention deficit behaviour in middle childhood and cannabis use by age 15. *Australian and New Zealand Journal of Psychiatry, 27*, 673–682.

Fergusson, D. M., Horwood, L. J. & Lynskey, M. T. (1994a). Parental separation. Adolescent psychopathology, and problem behaviors. *Journal of the American Academy of Child and Adolescent Psychiatry, 338*, 1122–1131.

Fergusson, D. M., Horwood, L. J. & Lynskey, M. T. (1994b). The comorbidities of adolescent problem behaviors. A latent class model. *Journal of Abnormal Child Psychology, 22*, 339–353.

Fergusson, D. M., Horwood, L. J. & Lynskey, M. T. (1994c). The childhoods of multiple problem adolescents: a 15-year longitudinal study. *Journal of Child Psychology and Psychiatry, 35*, 1123–1140.

Fergusson, D. M., Lynskey, M. T. & Horwood, L. J. (1994d). Childhood exposure to alcohol and adolescent drinking patterns. *Addiction, 89*, 1007–1016.

Fergusson, D. M., Boden, J. M. & Horwood L. J. (2006). Cannabis use and other illicit drug use: testing the cannabis gateway hypothesis. *Addiction, 101*, 556–569.

Ferri, M., Bargagli, A. M., Faggiano, F. *et al.* (2007). Mortality of drug users attending public treatment centers in Italy 1998–201: a cohort study. *Epidemiologia e Preventione, 31*, 276–282.

Fineschi, V. & Masti, A. (1996). Poisoning by MDMA (ecstasy) and MDEA: a case report. *International Journal of Legal Medicine, 108*, 272–275.

Firoz, S. & Carlson, G. (2004). Characteristics and treatment outcome of older methadone-maintenance patients. *American Journal of Geriatric Psychiatry, 12*, 539–541.

Fischer, B., Brissette, S., Brochu, S. *et al.* (2004). Determinants of overdose incidents among illicit opioid users in 5 Canadian cities. *Canadian Medical Association Journal, 171*, 235–239.

Fite, P. J., Wynn, P., Lochman, J. E. & Wells, K. C. (2009). The influence of neighborhood disadvantage and perceived disapproval on early substance use initiation. *Addictive Behaviors, 34*, 769–771.

Fleming, J. Mullen, P. E., Sibthorpe, B., Attewell, R. & Bammer, G. (1998). The relationship between childhood sexual abuse and alcohol abuse in women – a case-control study. *Addiction, 93*, 1787–1798.

Flynn, P. M., Joe, G. W., Broome, K. M., Simpson, D. D. & Brown, B. S. (2003). Recovery from opioid addiction in DATOS. *Journal of Substance Abuse Treatment, 25*, 177–186.

Forrester, M. B. (2007). Oxycodone abuse in Texas, 1998–2004. *Toxicology and Environmental Health, 70*, 534–538.

Foxcroft, D., Ireland, D., Lister-Sharp, D., Lowe, G. & Breen, R. (2003). Longer-term primary prevention for alcohol misuse in young people: a systematic review. *Addiction, 98*, 397–411.

Freeman, R. C., Parillo, K. M., Collier, K. & Rusek, R. W. (2001). Child and adolescent sexual abuse history in a sample of 1,490 women sexual partners of injection drug-using men. *Women and Health*, *34*, 31–49.

Friedman, L.S., Hyman, S. E. & Fleming, N. (1996). *Source Book of Substance Abuse and Addiction*. Maryland: Williams & Wilkins.

Fugelstad, A., Rajs, J., Bottiger, M., Gehrardsson, M. & de Verdier, M. G. (1995). Mortality among HIV-infected intravenous addicts in Stockholm in relation to methadone treatment. *Addiction*, *90*, 711–716.

Fugelstad, A., Ahlner, J., Brandt, L. *et al.* (2003). Use of morphine and 6-monoacetylmorphine in blood for the evaluation of possible risk factors for sudden death in 192 heroin users. *Addiction*, *98*, 463–470.

Fugelstad, A., Stenbacka, M., Leifman, A., Nylander, M. & Thiblin, I. (2007). Methadone maintenance treatment: the balance between life-saving treatment and fatal poisonings. *Addiction*, *102*, 406–412.

Fuller, C. M., Vlahov, D., Ompad, D. C., Shah, N., Arria, A. & Strathdee, S. A. (2002). High-risk behaviours associated with transition from illicit non-injection to injection drug use among adolescent and young adult drug users: a case-control study. *Drug and Alcohol Dependence*, *66*, 189–198.

Gable, R. S. (1993). Toward a comparative overview of dependence potential and acute toxicity of psychoactive substances used non-medically. *American Journal of Drug and Alcohol Abuse*, *19*, 263–281.

Galea, S., Ahern, J., Vlahov, D. *et al.* (2003). Income distribution and risk of fatal overdose in New York City neighbourhoods. *Drug and Alcohol Dependence*, *70*, 139–178.

Galea, S., Nandi, V. V. & Vlahov, D. (2004). The social epidemiology of substance use. *Epidemiologic Reviews*, *26*, 36–52.

Galea, S., Worthington, N., Piper, T. M., Nandi, V. V., Curtis, M. & Rosenthal, D. M. (2006). Provision of naloxone to injection drug users as an overdose prevention strategy: early evidence from a pilot study in New York City. *Addictive Behaviors*, *31*, 907–912.

Garofalo, R., Wolf, R. C., Kessel, S., Palfrey, J. & DuRant, R. H. (1998). The association between health risk behaviors and sexual orientation among a school-based sample of adolescents. *Pediatrics*, *101*, 895–902.

Gelkopf, M., Bleich, A., Hayward, R., Dodner, G., Adelson, M. (1999). Characteristics of benzodiazepine abuse in methadone maintenance treatment patients: a 1 year prospective study in an Israeli clinic. *Drug and Alcohol Dependence*, *55*, 63–68.

Gerstley, L. J., Alterman, A. I., McLellan, A. T., & Woody, G. E. (1990). Antisocial personality disorder in patients with substance abuse disorders: a problematic diagnosis?, *American Journal of Psychiatry*, *147*, 173–178.

Ghitza, U. E., Epstein, D. H. & Preston, K. L. (2008). Self-report of illicit benzodiazepine use on the Addiction Severity Index predicts treatment outcome. *Drug and Alcohol Dependence*, *97*, 150–157.

Gibbs, S. J., Beautrais A. L. & Fergusson, D. M. (2005). Mortality and further suicidal behaviour after an index suicide attempt: a 10-year study. *Australian and New Zealand Journal of Psychiatry*, *39*, 95–100.

Gibson, A. & Degenhardt, L. (2007). Mortality related to pharmacotherapies for opioid dependence: a comparative analysis of coronial records. *Drug and Alcohol Review*, *26*, 405–410.

Gibson, A. & Ritter, A. (2009). Naltrexone maintenance treatment. In R. P. Mattick, R. Ali. & N. Lintzeris. (eds.) *Pharmacotherapies for the Treatment of Opioid Dependence. Efficacy, Cost-effectiveness, and Implementation Guidelines*, pp. 252–281. New York: Informa Healthcare.

Gibson, D., Flynn, N. & Perales, D. (2001). Effectiveness of syringe exchange programs in reducing HIV risk behaviour and HIV seroconversion among injecting drug users. *AIDS*, *15*, 1329–1341.

Gilbert, L., El-Bassel, N., Schilling, R. F. & Friedman, E. (1997). Childhood abuse as a risk for partner abuse among women in methadone maintenance. *American Journal of Drug and Alcohol Abuse*, *23*, 581–595.

Gill, J. R. (2001). Fatal descent from height in New York City. *Journal of Forensic Sciences*, *46*, 1132–1137.

Gill, J. R. & Catanese, C. (2002). Sharp injury fatalities in New York City. *Journal of Forensic Sciences*, *47*, 554–557.

Gil-Rivas, V., Fiorentine, R., Anglin, M. D. & Taylor, E. (1997). Sexual and physical abuse: do they compromise drug treatment outcomes? *Journal of Substance Abuse Treatment*, *14*, 351–358.

Glatt, S., Bousman, C., Wang, R. *et al.* (2007). Evaluation of OPRM1 variants in heroin dependence by family-based association testing and meta-analysis. *Drug and Alcohol Dependence*, *90*, 159–165.

Goddard, E. (2008). *General Household Survey 2006: Smoking and Drinking among Adults*. London: Office for National Statistics.

Godfrey, C., Stewart, D. & Gossop, M. (2004). Economic analysis of costs and consequences of the treatment of drug misuse: 2-year outcome data from the National Treatment Outcome Research Study (NTORS). *Addiction*, *99*, 697–707.

Goldberg, R. J. & Grabowski, R. (2003). Methadone maintenance: its future in skilled nursing facilities. *Journal of the American Medical Directors Association*, *4*, 98–100.

Goldman, D., Oroszi, G. & Ducci, F. (2005). The genetics of addictions: uncovering the genes. *Nature Reviews Genetics*, *6*, 521–532.

Goldstein, A. & Herrara, J. (1995). Heroin addicts and methadone treatment in Albuquerque: a 22-year follow-up. *Drug and Alcohol Dependence*, *40*, 139–150.

Goldstein, P. J. (1985). The drugs/violence nexus: a tripartite conceptual framework. *Journal of Drug Issues*, *14*, 493–506.

Golub, A. & Johnson, B. D. (2002). Substance use progression and hard drug use in inner-city New York. In D. B. Kandel. (ed.) *Stages and Pathways of Drug*

Involvement. Examining the Gateway Hypothesis, pp. 90–114. Cambridge: Cambridge University Press.

Goodman, L. S. & Gilman, A. G. (1996). *Goodman and Gilman's The Pharmacological Basis of Therapeutics*, 9th edn. New York: McGraw Hill.

Goodwin, R. D., Fergusson, D. M. & Horwood, L. J. (2004). Association between anxiety disorders and substance use disorders among young persons: results of a 21-years longitudinal study. *Journal of Psychiatric Research*, *38*, 295–304.

Goren, N. (2005). *Social Marketing: Prevention and Practice Review*. Melbourne: Centre for Youth Drug Studies, Australian Drug Foundation.

Gossop, M. & Moos, R. (2008). Substance misuse among older adults: a neglected but treatable problem. *Addiction*, *103*, 347–348.

Gossop, M., Bradley, B. & Phillips, G. T. (1987). An investigation of withdrawal symptoms shown by opiate addicts during and subsequent to a 21-day inpatient methadone detoxification procedure, *Addictive Behaviors*, *12*, 1–6.

Gossop, M., Griffiths, P., Powis, B. & Strang, J. (1992). Severity of dependence and route of administration of heroin, cocaine and amphetamines. *British Journal of Addiction*, *87*, 1527–1536.

Gossop, M, Griffiths, P, Powis, B, Williamson, S. & Strang, J. (1996). Frequency of non-fatal heroin overdose: survey of heroin users recruited in non-clinical settings. *British Medical Journal*, *313*, 402.

Gossop, M., Marsden, J., Stewart, D. *et al.* (1998). Substance use, health and social problems of service users at 54 drug treatment agencies: intake data from the national treatment outcome research study. *British Journal of Psychiatry*, *193*, 166–171.

Gossop, M., Marsden, J., Stewart, D. & Rolfe, A. (1999). Treatment retention and 1 year outcomes for residential programmes in England. *Drug and Alcohol Dependence*, *57*, 89–98.

Gossop, M., Marsden, J., Stewart, D. & Rolfe, A. (2000). Patterns of improvement after methadone treatment: 1 year's follow-up results from the National Treatment Outcome Research Study. *Drug and Alcohol Dependence*, *60*, 275–286.

Gossop, M., Marsden, J., Stewart, D. & Treacy, S. (2002a). Change and stability of change after treatment of drug misuse. 2 year outcomes from the National Treatment Outcome Research Study. *Addictive Behaviours*, *27*, 155–166.

Gossop, M., Steward, D., Treacy, S. & Marsden, J. (2002b). A prospective study of mortality among drug misusers during a four year period after seeking treatment. *Addiction*, *97*, 39–47.

Graham, H. & Power, C. (2004). Childhood disadvantage and health inequalities: a framework for policy based on lifecourse research. *Child Care: Health and Development*, *30*, 671–678.

Grant, B. F. & Dawson, D. A. (1998). Age of onset and its association with DSM-IV drug abuse and dependence: results form the National Longitudinal Alcohol Epidemiological Survey. *Journal of Substance Abuse*, *10*, 163–173.

Grau, L. E., Dasgupta, N., Harvey, A. P. *et al.* (2007). Illicit use of opioids: is oxycontin a 'Gateway Drug'? *The American Journal on Addictions, 16,* 166–173.

Greenberg, M., Hamilton, R. & Toscano, G. (1999). Analysis of toxicology reports from the 1993–1994 census of fatal occupational injuries. *Compensation and Working Conditions, 4,* 26–28.

Griffiths, P., Gossop, M., Powis, B. & Strang, J. (1994). Transitions in patterns of heroin administration: a study of heroin chasers and injectors. *Addiction, 89,* 301–309.

Guichard A., Lert F., Calderon C. *et al.* (2003). Illicit drug use and injection practices among drug users on methadone and buprenorphine maintenance treatment in France. *Addiction, 98,* 1585–1597.

Gutierrez-Cebollada, J., De La Torre, R., Ortuno, J., Garces, J. & Cami, J. (1994). Psychotropic drug consumption and other factors associated with heroin overdose. *Drug and Alcohol Dependence, 35,* 169–174.

Haarstrup, S. & Jepson, P. W. (1988). Eleven year follow-up of 300 young opioid addicts. *Acta Psychiatrica Scandinavia, 77,* 22–26.

Haasen, C., Verthein, U., Degkwitz, P., Berger, J., Krausz, M. & Naber, D. (2007). Heroin-assisted treatment for opioid dependence randomised controlled trial. *British Journal of Psychiatry, 191,* 55–62.

Hagan, H., Des Jarlais, D. C., Stern, R. *et al.* (2007). HCV Synthesis Project: preliminary analyses of HCV prevalence in relation to age and duration of injection. *International Journal of Drug Policy, 18,* 341–351.

Hahesy, A. L., Wilens, T. E., Biederman, J., Van Patten, S. L. & Spencer, T. (2002). Temporal association between childhood psychopathology and substance. *Psychiatry Research, 109,* 245–253.

Haile, C. N., Kosten, T. A. & Kosten, T. R. (2008). Pharmacogenetic treatments for drug addiction: alcohol and opiates. *American Journal of Drug and Alcohol Abuse, 34,* 355–381.

Hall, W., Bell, J. & Carless, J. (1993). Crime and drug use among applicants for methadone maintenance. *Drug and Alcohol Dependence, 31,* 123–129.

Hall, W., Johnston, L. & Donnelly, N. (1999). Epidemiology of cannabis use and its consequences. In H. Kalant, W. Corrigall, W. Hall & R. Smart. (eds.) *The Health Effects of Cannabis,* pp. 71–125. Toronto: Centre for Addiction and Mental Health.

Hallinan, R., Byrne, A., Amin, J. & Dore, G. J. (2005). Hepatitis C virus prevalence and outcomes among injecting drug users on opioid replacement therapy. *Journal of Gastroenterology and Hepatology, 20,* 1082–1086.

Hamilton, A. B. & Grella, C. E. (2009). Gender differences among older heroin users. *Journal of Women and Aging, 21,* 111–124.

Harned, M. S., Najavitis, L. M. & Weiss, R. D. (2006). Self-harm and suicidal behaviour in women with comorbid PTSD and substance dependence. *The American Journal on Addictions, 15,* 392–5.

Harris, E. C. & Barraclough, B. (1997). Suicide as an outcome for mental disorders. *British Journal of Psychiatry, 170,* 205–228.

Harris, E. C. & Barraclough, B. (1998). Excess mortality of mental disorder. *British Journal of Psychiatry*, *173*, 11–53.

Hartel, D. M., Schoenbaum, E. E., Lo, Y. & Klein, R. S. (2006). Gender differences in illicit substance use among middle-aged drug users with or at risk for HIV infection. *Clinical and Infectious Dieases*, *43*, 525–531.

Hartnoll, R. L., Mitcheson, M. C., Battersby, A. *et al.* (1980). Evaluation of heroin maintenance in controlled trial. *Archives of General Psychiatry*, *37*, 877–884.

Harwood, H., Fountain, D. & Livermore, G. (1998). *Economic Costs of Alcohol and Drug Abuse in the United States, 1992*. Bethesda MD: National Institutes of Health.

Hassan, R. (1995). *Suicide Explained. The Australian Experience*. Melbourne: Melbourne University Press.

Hatzitaskos, P., Soldatos, C. R., Kokkevi, A. & Stefanis, C. N. (1999). Substance abuse patterns and their association with psychopathology and type of hostility in male patients with borderline and antisocial personality disorder. *Comprehensive Psychiatry*, *40*, 278–282.

Hawkins, J., Catalano, R. & Miller, J. (1992). Risk and protective factors for alcohol and other drug problems in adolescence and early adulthood: implications for substance abuse prevention. *Psychological Bulletin*, *112*, 64–105.

Havard, A., Teesson, M., Darke, S. & Ross, J. (2006). Depression among heroin users: 12 month outcomes from the Australian Treatment Outcome Study (ATOS). *Journal of Substance Abuse Treatment*, *30*, 355–362.

Heffernan, K., Cloitre, M., Tardiff, K., Marzuk, P., Portera, L. & Leon, A. (2000). Childhood trauma as a correlate of lifetime opiate use in psychiatric patients. *Addictive Behaviors*, *25*, 797–803.

Hemmingsson, T., Lundberg, I., Romelsjo, A. & Alfredsson, L. (1997). Alcoholism in social classes and occupations in Sweden. *International Journal of Epidemiology*, *26*, 584–591.

Hemstrom, O. (2002). Alcohol-related deaths contribute to socioeconomic differentials in mortality in Sweden. *European Journal of Public Health*, *12*, 254–262.

Henry, B., Feehan, M., McGee, R., Stanton, W., Moffitt, T. & Silva, P. (1993). The importance of conduct problems and depressive symptoms in predicting adolescent substance use. *Journal of Abnormal Child Psychology*, *21*, 469–480.

Herbert, J. R., Nichols, S. E. & Kabat, G. C. (1990). Indicators of nutritional status among clients from a New York City methadone treatment center. *Journal of Substance Abuse Treatment*, *7*, 161–165.

Hickman, M., Madden, P., Henry, J. *et al.* (2003). Trends in drug overdose deaths in England and Wales 1993–1998: methadone does not kill more people than heroin. *Addiction*, *98*, 419–425.

Hien, D. A., Nunes, E., Levin, F. R. & Fraser, D. (2000). Posttraumatic stress disorder and short-term outcome in early methadone treatment. *Journal of Substance Abuse Treatment*, *19*, 31–37.

Hoda, Z., Kerr, T., Li, K., Montaner, J. S. G. & Wood, E. (2008). Prevalence and correlates of jugular injections among injection drug users. *Drug and Alcohol Review, 27,* 442–446.

Hodgins, S., Cree, A., Alderton, J. & Mak, T. (2008). From conduct disorder to severe mental illness: associations with aggressive behaviour, crime and victimization. *Psychological Medicine, 38,* 975–987.

Horwood, L. J., Fergusson, D. M., Hayatbakhsh, M. R. *et al.* (2010). Cannabis use and educational achievement: findings from three Australasian cohort studies. *Drug and Alcohol Dependence, 110,* 247–253.

Hser, Y. (2007). Predicting long-term stable recovery from heroin addiction: findings from a 33-year follow-up. *Journal of Addictive Diseases, 26,* 51–60.

Hser, Y., Grella, C., Chou, C. P. & Anglin, M. D. (1998). Relationship between drug treatment careers and outcomes: findings from the National Drug Abuse Treatment Outcome Study. *Evaluation Review, 22,* 496–519.

Hser, Y., Grella, C. E., Hsieh, S., Anglin, M. D. & Brown, B. S. (1999). Prior treatment experience related to process and outcomes in DATOS. *Drug and Alcohol Dependence, 57,* 137–150.

Hser, Y., Hoffman, V., Grella, C. & Anglin, M. D. (2001). A 33-year follow-up of narcotic addicts. *Archives of General Psychiatry, 58,* 503–508.

Hser, Y., Gelberg, L., Hoffman, V. *et al.* (2004). Health conditions among aging narcotics addicts: medical examination results. *Journal of Behavioral Medicine, 27,* 607–622.

Hser, Y., Hunag, D., Chou, C. & Anglin, M. D. (2007a). Trajectories of heroin addiction. Growth mixture modelling results based on a 33-year follow-up study. *Evaluation Review, 6,* 548–563.

Hser, Y., Longshore, D. & Anglin, M. D. (2007b). The life course perspective on drug use: a conceptual framework for understanding drug use trajectories. *Evaluation Review, 6,* 515–547.

Hubbard, R. L., Marsden, M., Rachal, J., Harwood, H., Cavanaugh, E. & Ginzburg, H. (1989). *Drug Abuse Treatment: A National Study of Effectiveness.* Chapel Hill: University of North Carolina Press.

Hubbard R. L., Craddock, S. G., Flynn, P. M., Anderson, J. & Etheridge, R. M. (1997). Overview of one year follow-up outcomes in the Drug Abuse Treatment Outcome Study (DATOS). *Psychology of Addictive Behaviours, 11,* 261–278.

Humeniuk, R., Ali, R., McGregor, C. & Darke, S. (2003). Prevalence and correlates of intravenous methadone syrup administration in Adelaide, Australia. *Addiction, 98,* 413–418.

Inciardi, J. A. & Harrison, L. D. (eds.) (1998). *Heroin in the Age of Crack-Cocaine.* CA: Sage Publications.

Jenkinson R., Clark N. C., Fry C. L. & Dobbin M. (2005). Buprenorphine diversion and injection in Melbourne, Australia: an emerging issue? *Addiction, 100,* 197–205.

Joe, G. W. & Simpson, D. D. & Broome, K. M. (1998). Effects of readiness to change for drug abuse treatment on client retention and assessment of process. *Addiction*, *93*, 1177–1190.

Joe, G. W., Broome, K. M. & Simpson, D. D. (1999). Retention and patient engagement in models for different treatment modalities in DATOS. *Drug and Alcohol Dependence*, *57*, 113–125.

Johnson, R. A. & Gerstein, D. R. (1998). Initiation of use of alcohol, cigarettes, marijuana, cocaine, and other substances in US birth cohorts since 1919. *American Journal of Public Health*, *88*, 27–33.

Johnson, R. A. & Gerstein, D. R. (2000). Age, period, and cohort effects in marijuana and alcohol incidence: United States females and males, 1961–1990. *Substance Use and Misuse*, *35*, 925–948.

Johnsson, E. & Fridell, M. (1997). Suicide attempts in a cohort of drug abusers: a five year follow-up study. *Acta Psychiatrica Scandinavia*, *96*, 362–366.

Johnston, A., Pirkis, J. & Burgess, P. M. (2009). Suicidal thoughts and behaviours among Australian adults: findings from the 2007 National Survey of Mental Health and Wellbeing. *Australian and New Zealand Journal of Psychiatry*, *43*, 635–643.

Kakkoa, J., Heiliga, M. & Sarman, I. (2008). Buprenorphine and methadone treatment of opiate dependence during pregnancy: comparison of fetal growth and neonatal outcomes in two consecutive case series. *Drug and Alcohol Dependence*, *96*, 69–78.

Kalyoncu, A., Mırsal, H., Pektaş, O., Tan, D. & Beyazyürek, M. (2007). Heroin-dependent patients attempting and not attempting suicide: a comparison. *Acta Neuropsychiatrica*, *19*, 297–303.

Kandel, D. (1975). Sequences and stages in adolescent drug use. *Science*, *190*, 912–914.

Kandel, D. B. (1984). Marijuana users in young adulthood. *Archives of General Psychiatry*, *41*, 200–209.

Kandel, D. (1991). The social demography of drug use. *Milbank Quarterly*, *69*, 365–414.

Kandel, D. B. (ed.) (2002). *Stages and Pathways of Drug Involvement: Examining the Gateway Hypothesis*. Cambridge: Cambridge University Press.

Kandel, D. B. & Yamaguchi, K. (1999). Developmental stages of involvemnt in substance use. In R. E. Tarter, R. T. Ammerman & P. Ott. *Sourcebook on Substance Abuse: Etiology, Epidemiology, Assessment, and Treatment*, pp. 50–74. Needham: Alleyn & Bacon.

Kandel, D. B. & Yamaguchi, K. (2002). Stages of drug involvement in the US population. In D. B. Kandel. (ed.) *Stages and Pathways of Drug Involvement. Examining the Gateway Hypothesis*, pp. 65–89. Cambridge: Cambridge University Press.

Kandel D. B., Yamaguchi K. & Chen K. (1992). Stages of progression in drug involvement from adolescence to adulthood: further evidence for the gateway theory. *Journal of Studies on Alcohol*, *53*, 447–457.

Kandel, D., Chen, K., Warner, L. A., Kessler, R. C. & Grant, B. (1997). Prevalence and demographic correlates of symptoms of last year dependence on alcohol, nicotine, marijuana and cocaine in the US population. *Drug & Alcohol Dependence, 44*, 11–29.

Kanof, P. D., Aronson, M. J. & Ness, R. (1993). Organic mood syndrome associated with detoxification from methadone maintenance. *American Journal of Psychiatry, 150*, 423–428.

Karch, S. B. (2009). *Karch's Pathology of Drug Abuse,* 4th edn. Boca Raton: CRC Press.

Kaye, S., Darke, S. & Finlay-Jones, R. (1998). The onset of heroin use and criminal behaviour: does order make a difference? *Drug and Alcohol Dependence, 53*, 79–86.

Kaye, S., McKetin, R., Duflou, J. & Darke, S. (2007). Methamphetamine and cardiovascular pathology: a review of the evidence. *Addiction, 102*, 1204–1211.

Kelly, E., Darke, S. & Ross, J. (2004). A review of drug use and driving: epidemiology, impairment, risk factors and risk perceptions. *Drug and Alcohol Review, 23*, 319–344.

Kelly, T. M., Cornelius, J. R. & Clark, D. B. (2004). Psychiatric disorders and attempted suicide among adolescents with substance use disorders. *Drug and Alcohol Dependence, 73*, 87–97.

Kendler, K. S. & Prescott, C. A. (1998). Cocaine use, abuse and dependence in a population-based sample of female twins. *British Journal of Psychiatry, 173*, 345–350.

Kendler, K. S., Jacobson, K. C., Prescott, C. A. & Neale, M. C. (2003). Specificity of genetic and environmental risk factors for use and abuse/dependence of cannabis, cocaine, hallucinogens, sedatives, stimulants, and opiates in male twins. *American Journal of Psychiatry, 160*, 687–695.

Kerr, T., Oleson, M., Tyndall, M. W., Montaner, J. & Wood, E. (2005). A description of a peer-run supervised injection site for injecting drug users. *Journal of Urban Health: Bulletin of the New York Academy of Medicine, 82*, 267–275.

Kerr, T., Fairbairn, N., Tyndall, M. *et al.* (2007). Predictors of non-fatal overdose among a cohort of polysubstance-using injection drug users. *Drug and Alcohol Dependence, 87*, 39–45.

Kessler, R. C. & Wang, P. S. (2008). The descriptive epidemiology of commonly occurring mental disorders in the United States. *Annual Review of Public Health, 29*, 15–129.

Kessler, R. C., Berglund, P., Demler, O., Jin, R., Merikangas, K. R. & Walters, E. E. (2005). Lifetime prevalence and age-of-onset distributions of DSM-IV disorders in the national comorbidity survey replication. *Archives of General Psychiatry, 62*, 593–602.

Khantzian, E. J. & Treece, C. (1985). DSM-III psychiatric diagnosis of narcotic addicts. *Archives of General Psychiatry, 42*, 1067–1071.

Kidorf, M., Disney, E. R., King, V. L., Neufeld, K., Beilenson, P. L. & Brooner, R. K. (2004). Prevalence of psychiatric and substance use disorders in opioid abusers in a community syringe exchange program. *Drug and Alcohol Dependence*, *74*, 115–122.

Kimber, J., MacDonald, M., Van Beek, I. *et al.* (2003). The Sydney Medically Supervised Injecting Centre: client characteristics and predictors of frequent attendance during the first 12 months of operation. *Journal of Drug Issues*, *33*, 639–648.

Kintz, P. (2001). Deaths involving buprenorphine: a compendium of French cases. *Forensic Science International*, *121*, 65–69.

Kirchmayer, U., Davoli, M., Verster, A. D., Amato, L., Ferri, M. & Perucci, C. A. (2002). A systematic review on the efficacy of naltrexone maintenance treatment in opioid dependence. *Addiction*, *97*, 1241–1249.

Knutson, J., DeGarmo, D. & Reid, J. (2004). Social disadvantage and neglectful parenting as precursors to the development of antisocial and aggressive child behavior: testing a theoretical model. *Aggressive Behavior*, *30*, 187–205.

Kosarac, B., Fox, A. A. & Collard, C. D. (2009). Effect of genetic factors on opioid action. *Current Opinion in Anaesthesiology*, *22*, 476–482.

Kotler, P. & Zaltman, G. (1971). Social marketing: an approach to planned social change. *Journal of Marketing*, *35*, 3–12.

Kral, A. H., Wenger, L., Carpenter, L., Wood, E., Kerr, T. & Bourgois, P. (2010). Acceptability of a safer injection facility among injection drug users in San Francisco. *Drug and Alcohol Dependence*, *110*, 160–163.

Kriegstein, A. R., Shungu, D. C., Millar, W. S. *et al.* (1999). Leukoencephalopathy and raised brain lactate from heroin vapor inhalation ("chasing the dragon"). *Neurology*, *53*, 1765–1773.

Kritz, S., Chu, M., John-Hull, C., Madray, C., Louie, B. & Brown, L. S. (2009). Opioid dependence as a chronic disease: the interrelationships between length of stay, methadone dose, and age on treatment outcome at an urban opioid treatment program. *Journal of Addictive Diseases, 28*, 53–56.

Kronstrand, R., Grundin, R. & Jonsson, J. (1998). Incidence of opiates, amphetamines, and cocaine in hair and blood in fatal cases of heroin overdose. *Forensic Science International*, *92*, 29–38.

Kunøe, N., Lobmaier, P., Vederhus, J. K. *et al.* (2009). Naltrexone implants after in-patient treatment for opioid dependence: randomised controlled trial. *The British Journal of Psychiatry*, *194*, 541–546.

Lachman, M., Fann, C. S. J., Bartzis, M. *et al.* (2007) Genomewide suggestive linkage of opioid dependence to chromosome 14q. *Human Molecular Genetics*, *16*, 1327–1334.

Laslett, A. M., Dietze, P. & Dwyer, R. (2008). The oral health of street-recruited injecting drug users: prevalence and correlates of problems. *Addiction*, *103*, 1821–1825.

Lau, J. T. F, Kim, J. H., Tsui, H. Y., Cheung, A., Lau, M. & Yu, A. (2005). The relationship between physical maltreatment and substance use among adolescents: a survey of 95,788 adolescents in Hong Kong. *Journal of Adolescent Health*, *37*, 110–119.

Lemstra, M., Bennett, N. R., Neudorf, C. *et al.* (2008). A meta-analysis of marijuana and alcohol use by socio-economic status in adolescents aged 10–15 years. *Canadian Journal of Public Health*, *99*, 172–177.

Lenton, S. R. & Hargreaves, K. M. (2000). Should we conduct a trial of distributing naloxone to heroin users for peer administration to prevent fatal overdose? *Medical Journal of Australia*, *173*, 260–263.

Lenton, S., Dietze, P., Degenhardt, L., Darke, S. & Butler, T. G. (2009). Now is the time to take steps to allow peer access for heroin overdose in Australia. *Drug and Alcohol Review*, *28*, 583–585.

Li, Y., Ye, L., Jin-Song, P. *et al.* (2007). Morphine inhibits intrahepatic interferon-α expression and enhances complete hepatitis C virus replication. *The Journal of Infectious Diseases*, *196*, 719–730.

Ling, W., Charuvastra, C., Collins, J. F. *et al.* (1998). Buprenorphine maintenance treatment of opiate dependence: a multicenter, randomized clinical trial. *Addiction*, *93*, 475–486.

Lintzeris, N., Mitchell, T. B., Bond, A. J., Nestor, L. & Strang, J. (2006). Interactions on mixing diazepam with methadone or buprenorphine in maintenance patients. *Journal of Clinical Psychopharmacology*, *26*, 274–283.

Lintzeris, N., Mitchell, T. B., Bond, A. J., Nestor, L. & Strang, J. (2007). Pharmacodynamics of diazepam co-administered with methadone or buprenorphine under high dose conditions in opioid dependent patients. *Drug and Alcohol Dependence*, *91*, 187–194.

Lintzeris, N., Gowing, L. & Bell, J. (2009). Services for heroin withdrawal. In R. P. Mattick., R. Ali & N. Lintzeris. (eds.) *Pharmacotherapies for the Treatment of Opioid Dependence. Efficacy, Cost-effectiveness, and Implementation Guidelines*, pp. 54–106. New York: Informa Healthcare.

Lipman, E. L., Boyle, M. H., Dooley, M. D. & Offord, D. R. (2002). Child well-being in single mother families. *Journal of the American Academy of Child and Adolescent Psychiatry*, *41*, 75–82.

Löbmann, R. & Verthein, U. (2009). Explaining the effectiveness of heroin-assisted treatment on crime reductions. *Law and Human Behavior*, *33*, 83–95.

Loeber, R., Southamer-Lober, M. & White, H. (1999) Developmental aspects of delinquency and internalising problems and their association with persistent juvenile substance use between ages 7 and 18. *Journal of Clinical Child Psychology*, *28*, 322–332.

Lofwall, M. R., Brooner, R. K., Bigelow, G. E., Kindbom, K. & Strain, E. C. (2005). Characteristics of older opioid maintenance patients. *Journal of Substance Abuse Treatment*, *28*, 265–272.

Lubman, D. I., Yücel, M. & Hall, W. D. (2007). Substance use and the adolescent brain: a toxic combination? *Journal of Psychopharmacology*, *21*, 794.

Lucas, J., Goldfeder, L. B. & Gill, J. R. (2002). Bodies found in the waterways of New York City. *Journal of Forensic Science, 47,* 137–141.

Luthar, S. S., Merikangas, K. R. & Rounsaville, B. J. (1993). Parental psychopathology and disorders in offspring. A study of relatives of drug abusers. *Journal of Nervous and Mental Disease, 181,* 351–357.

Luthar, S. S., Cushing, G. & Rounsaville, B. J. (1996). Gender differences among opioid abusers: pathways to disorder and profiles of psychopathology. *Drug and Alcohol Dependence, 43,* 179–189.

Luthar, S. S., Cicchetti, D. & Becker, B. (2000). The construct of resilience: a critical evaluation and guidelines for future work. *Child Development, 71,* 543–562.

Luty, J. S. (2003). Social problems, psychological well-being, and childhood parenting experiences in a community sample of heroin addicts in central London. *Substance Use and Misuse, 38,* 201–219.

Lynskey, M. T. & Fergusson, D. (1995). Childhood conduct problems, attention deficit behaviors, and adolescent alcohol, tobacco, and illicit drug use. *Journal of Abnormal Child Psychology, 23,* 281–301.

Lynskey, M. & Hall, W. (1998). Cohort trends in age of initiation to heroin use. *Drug and Alcohol Review, 3,* 289–297.

Lynskey, M. & Hall, W. (2000). The effects of adolescent cannabis use on educational attainment: a review. *Addiction, 95,* 1621–1630.

Lynskey, M. T., Fergusson, D. & Horwood, L. J. (1994). The effects of parental alcohol problems on rates of adolescent psychiatric disorders. *Addiction, 89,* 1277–1286.

Lynskey, M., Degenhardt, L. & Hall, W. (2000). Cohort trends in youth suicide in Australia. *Australian and New Zealand Journal of Psychiatry, 34,* 408–412.

Maher, L., Swift, W. & Dawson, M. (2001). Heroin purity and composition in Sydney, Australia. *Drug and Alcohol Review, 20,* 439–448.

Maher, L., Dixon, D., Hall, W. & Lynskey, M. (2002). Crime and income generation by heroin users. *Australian and New Zealand Journal of Criminology, 35,* 187–202.

Maloney, E., Degenhardt, L., Darke, S. & Nelson, E. C. (2009). Are non-fatal opioid overdoses misclassified suicide attempts? Comparing the associated correlates. *Addictive Behaviors, 34,* 723–729.

Maloney, E., Degenhardt, L., Darke, S. & Nelson, E. C. (2010). Investigating the co-occurrence of self-mutilation and suicide attempts among opioid dependent individuals. *Suicide and Life-Threatening Behavior, 40,* 50–62.

Man, L. H., Berst, D., Gossop, M., Noble, A. & Strang, J. (2002). Risk of overdose: do those who witness most overdoses also experience most overdoses? *Journal of Substance Use, 7,* 136–140.

Manfredi, R., Sabbatani, S. & Agostini, D. (2006). Trend of mortality observed in a cohort of drug addicts of the metropolitan area of Bologna, North-Eastern Italy, during a 25-year-period. *Collegium Antropologicum, 30,* 479–488.

Manzoni, P., Brochu, S., Fischer, B. & Rehm, J. (2006). Determinants of property crime among illicit opiate users outside of treatment across Canada. *Deviant Behavior*, *27*, 351–376.

Mark, T. L., Woody, G. E., Juday, T. & Kleber, H. D. (2001) The economic costs of heroin addiction in the United States. *Drug and Alchol Dependence*, *61*, 195–206.

Martyres, R. F., Clode, D. & Burns, J. M. (2004). Seeking drugs or seeking help? Escalating 'doctor shopping' by young heroin users before fatal overdose. *Medical Journal of Australia*, *180*, 211–214.

Marzuk, P., Tardiff, K., Leon, A. *et al.* (1997). Poverty and fatal accidental drug overdoses of cocaine and opiates in New York City: an ecological study. *American Journal of Drug and Alcohol Abuse*, *23*, 221–228.

Masten, A. S. & Obravidic, J. (2006). Competence and resilience in development. *Annals of the New York Academy of Sciences*, *1094*, 13–27.

Mathers, B., Degenhardt, L., Phillips, B. *et al.* (2008). Global epidemiology of injecting drug use and HIV among people who inject drugs: a systematic review. *The Lancet*, *372*, 1733–1745.

Mattick, R. P., Ali, R. & Lintzeris, N. (eds.) (2009). *Pharmacotherapies for the Treatment of Opioid Dependence. Efficacy, Cost-effectiveness, and Implementation Guidelines*. New York: Informa Healthcare.

Mayer, P. & Hollt, V. (2006). Pharmacogenetics of opioid receptors and addiction. *Pharmacogenetics and Genomics*, *16*, 1–7.

Maxwell, J. C., Pullum, T. W. & Tannert, K. (2005). Deaths of clients in methadone treatment in Texas, 1994–2002. *Drug and Alcohol Dependence*, *78*, 73–81.

McBride, N. (2003). A systematic review of school drug education. *Health Education Research: Theory and Practice*, *18*, 729–742.

McCool, R. M. & Richter, K. P. (2003). Why do so many drug users smoke? *Journal of Substance Abuse Treatment*, *25*, 43–49.

McGlothlin, W. H. & Anglin, M. D. (1981). Long-term follow-up of clients of high- and low-dose methadone programs. *Archives of General Psychiatry*, *38*, 1055–1063.

McGregor, C., Darke, S., Christie, P. & Ali, R. (1998). Experience of non-fatal overdose among heroin users in Adelaide: circumstances and risk perception. *Addiction*, *93*, 701–711.

McGregor, C., Ali, R., Christie, P. & Darke, S. (2001). Overdose among heroin users: evaluation of an intervention in South Australia. *Addiction Research*, *9*, 481–501.

McKetin, R., McLaren, J., Kelly, E., Lubman, D. & Hides, L. (2006). The prevalence of psychotic symptoms among methamphetamine users. *Addiction*, *101*, 1473–1478.

Meader, N. (2010). A comparison of methadone, buprenorphine and alpha2 adrenergic agonists for opioid detoxification: a mixed treatment comparison meta-analysis. *Drug and Alcohol Dependence*, *108*, 110–114.

Medina, K. L., Schweinsburg, A. D., Cohen-Zion, M., Nagel, B. J. & Tapert, S. F. (2007). Effects of alcohol and combined marijuana and alcohol use during adolescence on hippocampal volume and asymmetry. *Neurotoxicology and Tetratology, 29*, 141–152.

Medrano, M. A., Zule, W. A., Hatch, J. & Desmond, D. P. (1999). Prevalence of childhood trauma in a community sample of substance-abusing women. *American Journal of Drug and Alcohol Abuse, 25*, 449–462.

Miech, R., Chilcoat, H. & Harder, V. (2005). The increase in the association of education and cocaine use over the 1980s and 1990s: evidence for a 'historical period' effect. *Drug and Alcohol Dependence, 79*, 311–320.

Miller, C. L., Kerr, T., Strathdee, S. A., Li, K. & Wood, E. (2007). Factors associated with premature mortality among young injection drug users in Vancouver. *Harm Reduction Journal, 4*, 1–7.

Milloy, M. J. S., Kerr, T., Mathias, R. *et al.* (2008). Non-fatal overdose among a cohort of active injection drug users recruited from a supervised injection facility. *American Journal of Drug and Alcohol Abuse, 34*, 499–509.

Mills, K. L., Teesson, M., Darke, S., Ross, J. & Lynskey, M. (2004). Young people with heroin dependence: findings from the Australian Treatment Outcome Study (ATOS). *Journal of Substance Abuse Treatment, 27*, 67–73.

Mills, K., Lynskey, M., Teesson, M., Ross, J. & Darke, S. (2005). Post-traumatic stress disorder among people with heroin dependence in the Australian Treatment Outcome Study (ATOS): prevalence and correlates. *Drug and Alcohol Dependence, 77*, 243–249.

Minozzi, S., Amato, L., Vecchi, S., Davoli, M., Kirchmayer, U. & Verster, A. (2006). Naltrexone maintenance treatment for opioid dependence. *The Cochrane Database of Sytematic Reviews.* Jan 25; (1): CD001333.

Miotto, K., McCann, M. J., Rawson, R. A., Frosch, D. & Ling, W. (1997). Overdose, suicide attempts and death among a cohort of naltrexone-treated opioid addicts. *Drug and Alcohol Dependence, 45*, 131–134.

Molnar, B., Buka, S. & Kessler, R. (2001). Child sexual abuse and subsequent psychopathology: results from the National Comorbidity Survey. *American Journal of Public Health, 91*, 753–760.

Morgan, C. J., Muetzelfeldt, L., Muetzelfeldt, M., Nutt, D. J. & Curran, H. V. (2010). Harms associated with psychoactive substances: findings from the UK National Drug Survey. *Journal of Psychopharmacology, 24*, 147–153.

Morral, A. R., McCaffrey, D. F. & Paddock, S. M. (2002). Reassessing the marijuana gateway effect. *Addiction, 97*, 1493–1504.

Muntaner, C., Eaton, W. W., Dialai, C., Kessler, R. C. & Sorlie, P. D. (1998). Social class, assets, organizational control and the prevalence of common groups of psychiatric disorders. *Social Science and Medicine, 47*, 2043–2053.

Murray, C. J. L. & Lopez, A. D. (1997). Mortality by cause for eight regions of the world: Global Burden of Disease Study. *Lancet, 349*, 1269–1276.

Najman, J., Toloo, G. & Williams, G. M. (2008). Increasing socio-economic inequalities in drug-induced deaths in Australia: 1981–2002. *Drug and Alcohol Review*, 27, 613–618.

Nandi, A., Glass, T. A., Cole, S. R. (2010). Neighborhood poverty and injection cessation in a sample of injection drug users. *American Journal of Epidemiology*, 171, 391–398.

National Institute on Alcohol Abuse and Alcoholism. (2004/5). The effects of alcohol on physiological processes and biological development. *Alcohol Research and Health*, 28, 125–131.

Neaigus, A., Miller, M., Friedman, S. et al. (2001). Potential risk factors for the transition to injecting among non-injecting heroin users: a comparison of former injectors and never injectors. *Addiction*, 96, 847–860.

Neaigus, A., Gyermathy, A., Miller, M., Frajzngier, V. M., Friedman, S. R. & Des Jarlais, D. C. (2006). Transitions to injecting drug use amongst non-injecting heroin users. *Journal of Acquired Immune Deficiency Syndromes*, 41, 493–503.

Neale, J. & Robertson, M. (2005). Recent life problems and non-fatal overdose among heroin users entering treatment. *Addiction*, 100, 168–175.

Neale, J., Bloor, M. & Weir, C. (2005). Problem drug users and assault. *International Journal of Drug Policy*, 16, 393–402.

Newton, N., Andrews, G., Teesson, M., & Vogl, L. (2009). Delivering prevention for alcohol and cannabis using the internet: a cluster randomised controlled trial. *Preventive Medicine*, 48, 579–584.

Newton, N., Teesson, M., Vogl, L. & Andrews, G. (2010). Internet-based prevention for alcohol and cannabis use: final results of the Climate Schools course. *Addiction*, 105, 749–759.

Nixon, K. & McClain, J. A. (2010). Adolescence as a critical window for developing an alcohol use disorder: current findings in neuroscience. *Current Opinion in Psychiatry*, 23, 227–232.

Noble, A., Best, D., Man, L. H., Gossop, M. & Strang, J. (2002). Self-detoxification attempts among methadone maintenance patients: what methods and what success? *Addictive Behaviors*, 27, 575–584.

Nunes, E. V., Weissman, M. M., Goldstein, R. B. et al. (1998). Psychopathology of children of parents with opiate dependence and/or major depression. *Journal of the American Academy on Child and Adolescent Psychiatry*, 37, 1142–1151.

Nurco, D. N., Cisin, I. H. & Balter, M. B. (1981). Addict careers. I. A new typology. *International Journal of the Addictions*, 16, 1305–1325.

Nutt, D., King, L. A., Saulsbury, W. & Blakemore, C. (2007). Development of a rational scale to assess the harm of drugs of potential misuse. *Lancet*, 369, 1047–1053.

Nutt, D., King, L. A. & Phillips, L. D. (2010). Drug harms in the UK: a multicriteria analysis. *Lancet*, 376, 1558–1565.

Ochoa, K.C., Hahn, J. A., Seal, K. H. & Moss, A. R. (2001). Overdosing among young injection drug users in San Francisco. *Addictive Behaviors*, *26*, 453–460.

Ødegårda, E., Amundsena, E. J. & Kielland, K. B. (2007). Fatal overdoses and deaths by other causes in a cohort of Norwegian drug abusers – A competing risk approach. *Drug and Alcohol Dependence*, *89*, 176–182.

O'Driscoll, P. T., McGough, J., Hagan, H., Thiede, H., Critchlow, C. & Alexander, E. R. (2001). Predictors of accidental fatal drug overdose among a cohort of injection drug users. *American Journal of Public Health*, *91*, 984–987.

Office of Applied Studies. (2007). *2006 National Survey on Drug Use and Health*. Washington: US Department of Health and Human Services.

Oh, H., Yamazaki, Y. & Kawata, C. (1998). Prevalence and a drug use development model for the study of adolescent drug use in Japan. *Japanese Journal of Public Health*, *45*, 870–882.

Ohannessian, C. M., Hesselbrock, V. M., Kramer, J. *et al.* (2004). Parental substance use consequences and adolescent psychopathology. *Journal of Studies on Alcohol*, *65*, 725–730.

Oliver, P., Horspool, M. & Keen, J. (2005). Fatal opiate overdose following regimen changes in naltrexone treatment. *Addiction*, *100*, 560–561.

Ompad, D. C., Ikeda, R. M., Shah, N. *et al.* (2005). Childhood sexual abuse and age at initiation of injection drug use. *American Journal of Public Health*, *95*, 703–709.

Oppenheimer, E., Tobutt, C., Taylor, C. & Andrew, T. (1994). Death and survival in a cohort of heroin addicts from London clinics: a 22 year follow-up. *Addiction*, *89*, 1299–1308.

Orti, R. M., Domingo-Salvany, A., Munoz, A., MacFarlane, D., Suelves, J. M. & Anto, J. M. (1996). Mortality trends in a cohort of opiate addicts, Catalona, Spain. *International Journal of Epidemiology*, *25*, 545–553.

Ouimette, P., Kimerling, R., Shaw, J. & Moos, R. (2000). Physical and sexual abuse among women and men with substance use disorders. *Alcoholism Treatment Quarterly*, *18*, 7–17.

Oviedo-Joekes, E., Marchand, K., Guh, D. *et al.* (2011). History of reported sexual or physical abuse among long-term heroin users and their response to substitution treatment. *Addictive Behaviors*, *36*, 55–60.

Patterson, S., Lennings, C. J. & Davey, J. (2000). Methadone clients, crime, and substance use. *International Journal of Offender Therapy and Comparative Criminology*, *44*, 667–680.

Patton, G., Bond, L., Butler, H. & Glover, S. (2003). Changing schools, changing health? Design and implementation of the Gatehouse project. *Journal of Adolescent Health*, *33*, 231–239.

Paulozzi, L. J. (2006) Opioid analgesic involvement in drug abuse deaths in American metropolitan areas. *American Journal of Public Health*, *96*, 1755–1757.

Perez-Jimenez, J. P. & Robert, M. S. (1997). Transitions in the route of heroin use. *European Addiction Research*, *3*, 93–98.

Perkonigg, A., Pfister, H., Höfler, M. *et al.* (2006). Substance use and substance use disorders in a community sample of adolescents and young adults: incidence, age effects and patterns of use. *European Addiction Research, 12,* 187–196.

Perneger, T. V., Giner, F., del Rio, M. & Mino, A. (1998). Randomised trial of heroin maintenance programme for addicts who fail in conventional drug treatments. *British Medical Journal, 317,* 13–18.

Petronis K. R. & Anthony, J. C. (2003). A different kind of contextual effect: geographical clustering of cocaine incidence in the USA. *Journal of Epidemiology and Community Health, 57,* 893–900.

Phillips, G. T., Gossop, M. & Bradley, B. (1986). The influence of psychological factors on the opiate withdrawal syndrome. *British Journal of Psychiatry, 149,* 235–238.

Phillips, S., Matusko, J. & Tomasovic, E. (2007). Reconsidering the relationship between alcohol and lethal violence. *Journal of Interpersonal Violence, 1,* 66–84.

Plotzker, R. E., Metzger, D. S. & Holmes, W. C. (2007). Childhood sexual and physical abuse histories, PTSD, depression, and HIV risk outcomes in women injection drug users: a potential mediating pathway. *The American Journal on Addictions, 16,* 431–438.

Pollack, H. & Heimer, R. (2004). The impact and cost-effectiveness of methadone maintenance treatment in preventing HIV and hepatitis C. In J. Jager., W. Limburg., M. Kretzschmar., M. Postma & L. Wiessing. (eds.) *Hepatitis C and Injecting Drug Use: Impact, Costs and Policy Options.* EMCDDA Monograph 7, pp. 345–370. Luxembourg: Office for Official Publications of the European Communities.

Potterat, J. J., Rothenberg, R. B., Muth, S. Q., Darrow, W. W. & Phillips-Plummer, L. (1998). Pathways to prostitution: the chronology of sexual and drug abuse milestones. *Journal of Sex Research, 35,* 333–340.

Poulton, R., Caspi A., Milne B. J. *et al.* (2002). Association between children's experience of socioeconomic disadvantage and adult health: a life-course study. *Lancet, 360,* 1640–1645.

Powis, B., Griffiths, P., Gossop, M. & Strang, J. (1996). The differences between male and female drug users: community samples of heroin and cocaine users compared. *Substance Use and Misuse, 31,* 529–543.

Powis, B., Strang, J., Griffiths, P. *et al.* (1999). Self-reported overdose among injecting drug users in London: extent and nature of the problem. *Addiction, 94,* 471–478.

Preti, A., Miotto, P. & De Coppi, M. (2002). Deaths by unintentional illicit drug overdose in Italy, 1984–2000. *Drug and Alcohol Dependence, 66,* 275–282.

Prochaska, J. O. & Velicer, W. F. (1997). The transtheoretical model of health behavior change. *American Journal of Health, Promotion, 12,* 38–48.

Prochaska, J. O., DiClemente, C. C., Velicer, W. F., Ginpil, S. & Norcross, J. C. (1985). Predicting change in smoking status for self-changers. *Addictive Behaviors, 10,* 395–406.

Pugatch, D., Strong, L. L., Has, P. *et al.* (2001). Heroin use in adolescents and young adults admitted for drug detoxification. *Journal of Substance Abuse, 13*, 337–346.

Quaglio, G., Talamini, G., Lechi, A. *et al.* (2001). Study of heroin-related deaths in north-eastern Italy 1985–98 to establish main causes of death. *Addiction, 96*, 1127–1137.

Quan, V., Vongchak, T., Jittiwutikan, J. *et al.* (2007). Predictors of mortality among injecting and non-injecting HIV-negative drug users in northern Thailand. *Addiction, 102*, 441–446.

Rajaratnam, R., Sivesind, D., Todman, M., Roane, D. & Seewald, R. (2009). The aging methadone maintenance patient: treatment adjustment, long-term success, and quality of life. *Journal of Opioid Management, 5*, 27–37.

Rathod, N. H., Addenbrooke, W. M. & Rosenbach, A. F. (2005). Heroin dependence in an English town: 33-year follow-up. *British Journal of Psychiatry, 187*, 421–425.

Ravndal, E. & Amundsen, E. J. (2010). Mortality among drug users after discharge from inpatient treatment: an 8-year prospective study. *Drug and Alcohol Dependence, 108*, 65–69.

Ravndal, E., Lauritzen, G., Jansson, S. O., Larsson, J. (2001). Childhood maltreatment among Norwegian drug abusers in treatment. *International Journal of Social Welfare, 10*, 142–147.

Reece, A. S. (2007). Dentition of addiction in Queensland: poor dental status and major contributing drugs. *Australian Dental Journal, 52*, 144–149.

Reed, L. J., Glasper, A., de Wet, C. J., Bearn, J. & Gossop, M. (2007). Comparison of buprenorphine and methadone in the treatment of opiate withdrawal: possible advantages of buprenorphine for the treatment of opiate-benzodiazepine codependent patients? *Journal of Clinical Psychopharmacology, 27*, 188–192.

Rehm, J., Gschwend, P., Steffen, T., Gutzwiller, F., Dobler-Mikola, A. & Uchtenhagen, A. (2001). Feasibility, safety, and efficacy of injectable heroin prescription for refractory opioid addicts: a follow-up study. *The Lancet, 358*, 1417–1420. http://www.sciencedirect.com/science/journal/01406736358

Rehm, J., Frick, U., Hartwig, C., Gutzwiller, F., Gschwend, P. & Uchtenhagen, A. (2005). Mortality in heroin-assisted treatment in Switzerland 1994–2000. *Drug and Alcohol Dependence, 79*, 137–143.

Rehm, J., Baliunas, D., Brochu, S. *et al.* (2006). *The Cost of Subsance Abuse in Canada 2002*. Ottawa: Canadian Centre on Substance Abuse.

Risser, D., Uhl, A., Stichenwirth, M. *et al.* (2000). Quality of heroin and heroin-related deaths from 1987 to 1995 in Vienna, Austria. *Addiction, 95*, 375–382.

Roberts, A., Mathers, B., Howard, J. & Degenhardt, L. (2010). *Women Who Inject Drugs: A Review of their Risks, Experiences and Needs*. Sydney: University of New South Wales.

Robertson, J. R., Ronald, P. J. M., Raab, G., Ross, A. J. & Parpia, T. (1994). Deaths, HIV infection, abstinence, and other outcomes in a cohort of injecting drug users followed up for 10 years. *British Medical Journal, 309*, 369–372.

Robins, L. N. (1993). Vietnam veterans' rapid recovery from heroin addiction: a fluke or normal expectation? *Addiction, 88,* 1041–1054.

Rosen, D., Smith, M. L. & Reynolds, C. F. (2008). The prevalence of mental and physical health disorders among older methadone patients. *American Journal of Geriatric Psychiatry, 16,* 488–497.

Rosen, S., Ouimette, P. C., Sheikh, J. I., Gregg, J. A. & Moos, R. H. (2002). Physical and sexual abuse history and addiction treatment outcomes. *Journal of Studies on Alcohol, 63,* 683–687.

Ross, J. & Darke, S. (2000). The nature of benzodiazepine dependence among heroin users in Sydney, Australia. *Addiction, 95,* 1785–1793.

Ross, J., Darke, S. & Hall, W. (1997). Transitions between routes of benzodiazepine administration among heroin users in Sydney. *Addiction, 92,* 697–705.

Ross, J., Teesson, M., Darke, S., Lynskey, M., Ali, R., Ritter, A. & Cooke, R. (2005). The characteristics of heroin users entering treatment: findings from the Australian Treatment Outcome Study (ATOS). *Drug and Alcohol Review, 24,* 411–418.

Ross, J., Teesson, M., Darke, S., Lynskey, M., Ali, R., Ritter, A. & Cooke, R. (2006). Short-term outcomes for the treatment of heroin dependence: findings from the Australian Treatment Outcome Study (ATOS). *Addictive Disorders and Their Treatment, 5,* 133–144.

Rossow, I. (1994). Suicide among drug addicts in Norway. *Addiction, 89,* 1667–1673.

Rossow, I. & Lauritzen, G. (1999). Balancing on the edge of death: suicide attempts and life-threatening overdoses among drug addicts. *Addiction, 94,* 209–219.

Rossow, I. & Lauritzen, G. (2001). Shattered childhood: a key issue in suicidal behavior among drug addicts. *Addiction, 96,* 227–240.

Rothenberg, J. L., Sullivan, M. A., Church, S. H. *et al.* (2002). Behavioral naltrexone therapy: An integrated treatment for opiate dependence. *Journal of Substance Abuse Treatment, 23,* 351–360.

Rothman, R. A. & Stephens, R. S. (eds.) (2006). *Cannabis Dependence. Its Nature, Consequences and Treatment.* Cambridge: Cambridge University Press.

Rounsaville, B. J., Kosten, T. & Kleber, H. (1985). Success and failure at outpatient opioid detoxification: evaluating the process of clonidine- and methadone-assisted withdrawal. *Journal of Nervous and Mental Disease, 173,* 103–110.

Rouser, E., Brooner, R. K., Regier, M. W. & Bigelow, G. E. (1994). Psychiatric distress in antisocial drug abusers: relation to other personality disorders. *Drug Alcohol Dependence, 34,* 149–154.

Roxburgh, A., Hall, W. D., Degenhardt, L. *et al.* (2010). Trends in cannabis use and cannabis-related harm in Australia 1993–2007, *Addiction, 105,* 1071–1079.

Roy, A. (2002). Characteristics of opiate dependent patients who attempt suicide. *Journal of Clinical Psychiatry, 63,* 403–407.

Roy, A. (2010). Risk factors for attempting suicide in heroin addicts. *Suicide and Life-Threatening Behavior, 40,* 416–420.

Roy, E., Haley, N., Leclerc, P., Cédras, L. & Boivin, J-F. (2002). Drug injection among street youth: the first time. *Addiction*, *97*, 1003–1009.

Rutherford, M. J., Cacciola, J. S. & Alterman, A. I. (1994). Relationships of personality disorders with problem severity in methadone patients. *Drug and Alcohol Dependence*, *35*, 69–76.

Ruttenber, A. J. & Luke, J. L. (1984). Heroin-related deaths: new epidemiologic insights. *Science*, *226*, 14–20.

Ruttenber, A. J., Kalter, H. O. & Santinga, P. (1990). The role of ethanol abuse in the etiology of heroin-related death. *Journal of Forensic Sciences*, *35*, 891–900.

Salamina, G., Diecidue, R., Vigna-Taglianti, F. *et al.* (2010). Effectiveness of therapies for heroin addiction in retaining patients in treatment: results from the VEdeTTE study. *Substance Use and Misuse*, *45*, 2076–2092.

San, L., Pomarol, G., Peri, M., Olle, M. & Cami, J. (1991). Follow-up after a six-month maintenance period on naltrexone versus placebo in heroin addicts. *British Journal of Addiction*, *86*, 983–990.

Sanchez-Carbonell, J., Cami, J. & Brigo, S. B. (1988). Follow-up of heroin addicts in Spain (EMETYST project): results 1 year after treatment admission, *British Journal of Addiction*, *83*, 1439–1448.

Sanchez-Carbonell, X. & Seus, L. (2000). Ten-year survival analysis of a cohort of heroin addicts in Catalonia: the EMETYST project. *Addiction*, *95*, 941–948.

Sansone, R. A., Whitecar, P. & Wiederman, M. W. (2009). The prevalence of childhood trauma among those seeking buprenorphine treatment. *Journal of Addictive Diseases*, *28*, 64–67.

Santelli, J. S., Kaiser, J., Hirsch, L., Radosh, A., Simkin, L. & Middlestadt, S. (2004). Initiation of sexual intercourse among middle school adolescents: the influence of psychosocial factors. *Journal of Adolescent Health*, *34*, 200–208.

Saxon, A. J., Oreskovich, M. R., & Brkanac, Z. (2005). Genetic determinants of addiction to opioids and cocaine. *Harvard Review of Psychiatry 13*, 218–232.

Schaar, I. & Ojehagan, A. (2001). Severely ill substance abusers: an 18-month follow-up study. *Social Psychiatry and Psychiatric Epidemiology*, *36*, 70–78.

Scherbaum, N., Specka, M., Hauptmann, G. & Gastpar, M. (2002). Does maintenance treatment reduce the mortality rate of opioid addicts? *Fortschritte der Neurologie-Psychiatrie*, *70*, 455–61.

Schmittner, J., Schroeder, J. R., Epstein, D. H. & Preston, K. L. (2005). Menstrual cycle length during methadone maintenance. *Addiction*, *100*, 829–836.

Schmucker, D. L. (2005). Age-related changes in liver structure and function: implications for disease? *Experimental Gerontology*, *40*, 650–659.

Seal, K. H., Kral, A. H., Gee, L. *et al.* (2001). Prediction and prevention of non-fatal overdose among street-recruited injection heroin users in the San Francisco Bay area, 1998–1999. *American Journal of Public Health*, *91*, 1842–1846.

Seal, K. H., Thawley, R., Gee, L. *et al.* (2005). Naloxone distribution and cardiopulmonary resuscitaion training for injection drug users to prevent heroin overdose death: a pilot intervention. *Journal of Urban Health: Bulletin of the New York Academy of Medicine, 82*, 303–311.

Sergeev, B., Karpets, A., Sarang, A. & Tikhonov, M. (2003). Prevalence and circumstances of opiate overdose among injection drug users in the Russian federation. *Journal of Urban Health, 80*, 212–219.

Seymour, A., Black, M., Jay, J., Cooper, G., Weir, C. & Oliver, J. (2003). The role of methadone in drug-related deaths in the west of Scotland. *Addiction, 98*, 995–1002.

Sheehan, M., Oppenheimer, E. & Taylor, C. (1988). Who comes for treatment. Drug misusers at three London agencies. *British Journal of Addiction, 83*, 311–320.

Sheehan, M., Oppenheimer, E. & Taylor, C. (1993). Opiate users and the first years after treatment: outcome analysis of the proportion of follow-up time spent in abstinence. *Addiction, 88*, 1679–1689.

Shields, L. B. E., Hunsaker, D. M., Hunsaker, J. C. & Ward, M. K. (2006). Toxicologic findings in suicide. A 10-year retrospective review of Kentucky medical examiner cases. *American Journal of Forensic Medicine and Pathology, 27*, 106–112.

Shrier, L. A., Harris, S. K., Sternberg, M. & Beardslee, W. R. (2001). Associations of depression, self-esteem, and substance use with sexual risk among adolescents. *Preventive Medicine, 33*, 179–189.

Simini, B. (1998). Naloxone supplied to Italian heroin addicts. *The Lancet, 352*, 967.

Simpson, D. D. & Sells, S. B. (1982). Effectiveness of treatment for drug abuse: an overview of the DARP research program. *Advances in Substance Abuse, 2*, 27–29.

Simpson, D. D. & Sells, S. B. (eds.) (1990). *Opioid Addiction and Treatment: A 12-Year Follow-up*. Florida: Robert E. Kreiger Publishing.

Simpson, D. D., Joe, G. W. & Brown, B. S. (1997). Treatment retention and follow-up outcomes. The Drug Abuse Treatment Outcome Study (DATOS). *Psychology of Addictive Behaviors, 4*, 294–307.

Simons, L. & Giorgio, T. (2008). Characteristics of substance abusing men and women entering a drug treatment program. An exploration of sex differences. *Addictive Disorders and Their Treatment, 7*, 15–23.

Slade, T., Johnston, A., Browne, O., Andrews, G. & Whiteford, H. (2009). 2007 National Survey of Mental Health and Wellbeing: methods and key findings. *Australian and New Zealand Journal of Psychiatry, 43*, 594.

Smolka, M. & Schmidt, L. G. (1999). The influence of heroin dose and route of administration on the severity of the opiate withdrawal syndrome. *Addiction, 94*, 1191–1198.

Smyth, B. P., O'Brien, M. & Barry, J. (2000). Trends in treated opiate misuse in Dublin: the emergence of chasing the dragon. *Addiction, 95*, 1217–1223.

Smyth, B., Hoffman, V., Fan, J. & Hser, Y. (2007). Years of potential life lost among heroin addicts 33 years after treatment. *Preventative Medicine, 44*, 369–374.

Soyka, M., Apelt, S., Lieb, M. & Wittchen, H. (2006). One-year mortality rates of patients receiving methadone and buprenorphine maintenance therapy: a nationally representative cohort study in 2694 patients. *Journal of Clinical Psychopharmacology*, *26*, 657–660.

Spijkerman, I. J. B., Koot, M., Prins, M. *et al.* (1995). Lower prevalence and incidence of HIV-1 syncytium-inducing phenotype among injecting drug users compared with homosexual men. *AIDS*, *9*, 1085–1092.

Spittal, P. M., Bruneau, J., Craib, K. J. P. *et al.* (2003). Surviving the sex trade: a comparison of HIV risk behaviours among street-involved women in two Canadian cities who inject drugs. *AIDS Care*, *15*, 187–195.

Spooner, C. & Hetherington, K. (2005). *Social Determinants of Drug Use*. National Drug and Alcohol Research Centre Technical Report No. 228. Sydney: University of New South Wales.

Stafford, J., Sindicich, N., Burns, L. *et al.* (2008). *Australian Drug Trends 2008: Findings from the Illicit Drug Reporting System (IDRS)*. Australian Drug Trends Series No. 19. Sydney: National Drug and Alcohol Research Centre.

Stapleton, R. D. & Comiskey, C. M. (2010). Alcohol usage and associated treatment outcomes for opiate users entering treatment in Ireland. *Drug and Alcohol Dependence*, *107*, 56–61.

Stenbacka, M., Liefman, L. & Romelsjo, A. (2010). Mortality and cause of death among 1705 illicit drug users, a 37 year follow-up. *Drug and Alcohol Review 29*, 21–27.

Stewart, D., Gossop, M. & Marsden, J. (2002). Reductions in non-fatal overdose after drug misuse treatment: results from the National Treatment Outcome Research Study (NTORS). *Journal of Substance Abuse Treatment*, *22*, 1–9.

Stewart, L. M., Henderson, C. J., Hobbs, M. T., Ridout, S. C. & Knuiman, M. W. (2004). Risk of death in prisoners after release from jail. *Australian and New Zealand Journal of Public Health*, *28*, 32–36.

Strain, E. C., Stitzer, M. L. & Bigelow, G. E. (1991). Early treatment time course of depressive symptoms in opiate addicts. *Journal of Nervous and Mental Disease*, *179*, 215–221.

Strang, J., Griffiths, P. & Gossop, M. (1997). Heroin smoking by 'chasing the dragon': origins and history. *Addiction*, *92*, 673–683.

Strang, J., Griffiths, P., Powis, B. & Gossop, M. (1999a). Heroin chasers and heroin injectors: differences observed in a community sample in London, UK. *American Journal of the Addictions*, *8*, 148–160.

Strang, J., Powis, B., Best, D. *et al.* (1999b). Preventing opiate overdose fatalities with take-home naloxone: pre-launch study of possible impact and acceptability. *Addiction*, *94*, 199–204.

Strang, J., Best, D., Man, L. H., Noble, A. & Gossop, M. (2000). Peer-initiated resuscitation: fellow drug users could be mobilised to implement resuscitation. *International Journal of Drug Policy*, *11*, 437–445.

Strang, J., McCambridge, J., Best, D. *et al.* (2003). Loss of tolerance and overdose mortality after inpatient opiate detoxification: follow up study. *British Medical Journal, 356,* 959–960.

Strassels, S. A. (2009). Economic burden of prescription opioid misuse and abuse. *Journal of Managed Care Pharmacy, 15,* 556–562.

Stueve, A. & O'Donnell, L. N. (2005). Alcohol initiation and subsequent sexual and alcohol risk behaviors among urban youths. *American Journal of Public Health, 95,* 887–893.

Surratt, H. L., Inciardi, J. A., Kurtz, S. P. & Kiley, M. C. (2004). Sex work and drug use in a subculture of violence. *Crime and Delinquency, 50,* 43–59.

Swift, W., Maher, L., Sunjic, S. & Doan, V. (1999). Transitions between routes of heroin administration: a study of Caucasian and Indo-Chinese heroin users in south-western Sydney, Australia. *Addiction, 94,* 71–82.

Tagliaro, F., Debattisti, Z., Smith, F. P. & Marigo, M. (1998). Death from heroin overdose: findings from hair analysis. *Lancet, 351,* 1923–1925.

Tardiff, K., Wallace, Z., Tracy, M., Piper, T. M., Vlahov, D. & Galla, S. (2005). Drug and alcohol use as determinants of New York city homicide trends from 1990 to 1998. *Journal of Forensic Science, 50,* 470–474.

Teesson, M., Havard, A., Fairbairn, S., Ross, J., Lynskey, M. & Darke, S. (2005). Depression among entrants to treatment for heroin dependence in the Australian Treatment Outcome Study (ATOS): prevalence, correlates and treatment seeking. *Drug and Alcohol Dependence, 78,* 309–315.

Teesson, M., Havard, A., Ross, J. & Darke, S. (2006a). Outcomes after detoxification for heroin dependence: findings from the Australian Treatment Outcome Study (ATOS). *Drug and Alcohol Review, 25,* 241–247.

Teesson, M., Ross, J., Darke, S., Lynskey, M., Ali, R., Cooke, R. & Ritter, A. (2006b). The Australian Treatment Outcome Study (ATOS): 1 year follow-up results. *Drug and Alcohol Dependence, 83,* 174–180.

Teesson, M., Mills, K. L., Ross, J., Darke, S., Williamson, A. & Havard, A. (2008). The impact of treatment on 3 year outcomes for heroin dependence: findings from the Australian Treatment Outcome Study (ATOS). *Addiction, 103,* 80–88.

Teesson, M., Hall, W., Slade, T. *et al.* (in press). Prevalence and correlates of DSM-IV alcohol abuse and dependence in Australia: findings from the 2007 National Survey of Mental Health and Wellbeing. *Addiction.*

Termorshuizen, F., Krol, A., Prins, M. & van Ameijden, E. J. C. (2005). Long-term outcome of chronic drug use: the Amsterdam Cohort Study among drug users. *American Journal of Epidemiology, 161,* 271–279.

Tobler, N. & Stratton, H. (1997). Effectiveness of school-based drug prevention programs: a meta-analysis of the research. *Journal of Primary Prevention, 18,* 71–125.

Tobin, K. E. & Latkin, C. A. (2003). The relationship between depressive symptoms and non-fatal overdose among a sample of drug users in Baltimore, Maryland. *Journal of Urban Health*, *80*, 220–229.

Tobin, K. E., Davey, M. A. & Latkin, C. A. (2005). Calling emergency medical services during drug overdose: an examination of individual, social and setting correlates. *Addiction*, *100*, 397–404.

Torok, M., Darke, S., Kaye, S. & Ross, J. (in press). Conduct disorder as a risk factor for violent victimization and offending amongst regular illicit drug users. *Journal of Drug Issues*.

Trémeau, F. A. D., Staner, L., Corrêa, H. *et al.* (2008). Suicidality in opioid-dependent subjects. *The American Journal on Addictions*, *17*, 187–194.

Triffleman, E. G., Marmar, C. R., Delucchi, K. L. & Ronfeldt, H. (1995). Childhood trauma and posttraumatic stress disorder in substance abuse inpatients. *Journal of Nervous and Mental Disease*, *183*, 172–176.

Trull, T. J., Sher, K. J., Minks-Brown, C., Durbin, J. & Burr, R. (2000). Borderline personality disorder and substance use disorders: a review and integration. *Clinical Psychology Review*, *20*, 235–253.

Tucker, T. K., Ritter, A., Maher, C. & Jackson, H. (2004). Naltrexone maintenance for heroin dependence: uptake, attrition and retention. *Drug and Alcohol Review*, *23*, 299–309.

Turk, E. E. & Tsokos, M. (2004). Pathologic features of fatal falls from height. *American Journal of Forensic Medicine and Pathology*, *25*, 194–199.

Tyndall, M. W., Craib, K. J. P., Currie, S., Li, K., O'Shaughnessy, M. V. & Schechter, M. T. (2001). Impact of HIV infection on mortality in a cohort of injection drug users. *Journal of Acquired Immune Deficiency Syndromes*, *28*, 351–357.

Tyrfingsson, T., Thorgeirsson, T. E., Geller, F. *et al.* (2010). Addictions and their familiality in Iceland. *Annals of The New York Academy of Sciences*, *1187*, 208–217.

United Nations Office of Drug Control (2009). *World Illicit Drug Report 2009*. New York: United Nations Publications.

Vaillant, G. (1973). A 20 year follow-up of New York narcotic addicts. *Archives of General Psychiatry*, *29*, 237–241.

van Ameijden, E. J. C., van den Hoek, J. A. R., Hartgers, C. & Coutinho, R. A. (1994). Risk factors for the transition from non-injection to injection drug use and accompanying AIDS risk behavior in a cohort of drug users. *American Journal of Epidemiology*, *139*, 1153–1163.

van Amsterdam, J., Opperhuizen, A., Koeter, M. & van den Brink, W. (2010). Ranking the harm of alcohol, tobacco and illicit drugs for the individual and the population. *European Addiction Research*, *16*, 202–207.

van den Brink, W., Hendriks, V. M., Blanken, P., Koeter, M. W. J., van Zwieten, B. J. & van Ree, J. M. (2003). Medical prescription of heroin to treatment resistant heroin addicts: two randomised controlled trials. *British Medical Journal*, *327*, 310–315.

Van der Zanden, B. P., Dijkgraaf, M. G. Blanken, P., van Ree J. M. & van den Brink, W. (2007). Patterns of acquisitive crime during methadone maintenance treatment among patients eligible for heroin assisted treatment. *Drug and Alcohol Dependence*, *86*, 84–90.

Van Etten, M. L. & Anthony, J. C. (1999). Comparative epidemiology of initial drug opportunities and transitions to first use: marijuana, cocaine, hallucinogens and heroin. *Drug and Alcohol Dependence*, *54*, 117–125.

Van Gundy, K. & Rebellon, C. J. (2010). A life-course perspective on the 'Gateway Hypothesis'. *Journal of Health and Social Behavior*, *51*, 244–259.

van Os, J., Bak, M., Hanssen, M., Bijl, R. V., de Graaf, R. & Verdoux, H. (2002). Cannabis use and psychosis: a longitudinal population-based study. *American Journal of Epidemiology*, *156*, 319–327.

van Ours, J. C. (2003). Is cannabis a stepping-stone for cocaine? *Journal of Health Economics*, *22*, 539–554.

van Ours, J. & Williams, J. (2009). Why parents worry: initiation into cannabis use by youth and their educational attainment. *Journal of Health Economics*, *28*, 132–142.

Velleman, R., Templeton, L. & Copello, A. (2005). The role of the family in preventing and intervening with substance use and misuse: a comprehensive review of family interventions, with a focus on young people. *Drug and Alcohol Review*, *24*, 93–109.

Vidal-Trecan, G., Varescon-Pousson, I. & Boissonnas, A. (2002). Injection risk behaviors at the first and at the most recent injections among drug users. *Drug and Alcohol Dependence*, *66*, 107–109.

Vidal-Trecan, G., Varescon, I., Nabet, N. & Boissonnas, A. (2003). Intravenous use of prescribed sublingual buprenorphine tablets by drug users receiving maintenance therapy in France. *Drug and Alcohol Dependence*, *69*, 175–181.

Vimpani, G. (2005). Getting the mix right: family, community and social policy interventions to improve outcomes for young people at risk of substance misuse. *Drug and Alcohol Review*, *24*, 111–125.

Vlahov, D. & Junge, B. (1998). The role of needle exchange programs in HIV prevention. *Public Health Reports*, *113* (suppl 1), 75–80.

Vlahov, D., Wang, C., Galai, N. *et al.* (2004). Mortality risk among new onset injection drug users. *Addiction*, *99*, 946–954.

Vlahov, D., Galai, N., Safaeian, M. *et al.* (2005). Effectiveness of highly active antiretroviral therapy among injection drug users with late-stage human immunodeficiency virus infection. *American Journal of Epidemiology*, *161*, 999–1012.

Vlahov, D., Wang, C., Ompad, D. *et al.* (2008). Mortality risk among recent-onset injection drug users in five US cities. *Substance Use and Misuse*, *43*, 413–428.

Vogl, L., Teesson, M., Andrews, G., Bird, K., Steadman, B. & Dillon, P. (2009). A computerized harm minimization prevention program for alcohol misuse and related harms: randomized controlled trial. *Addiction*, *104*, 564–575.

Wahren, C. A., Brandt, L. & Allebeck, P. (1997). Has mortality in drug addicts increased? A comparison between hospitalized cohorts in Stockholm. *International Journal of Epidemiology*, *26*, 1219–1226.

Ward, J, Mattick, R. P. & Hall, W. (eds.) (1998). *Methadone Maintenance Treatment and Other Opioid Replacement Therapies*. Amsterdam: Harwood.

Warner, L. A., Kessler, R. C., Hughes, M., Anthony, J. C. & Nelson, C. B. (1995). Prevalence and correlates of drug use and dependence in the United States. Results from the National Comorbidity Survey. *Archives of General Psychiatry*, *52*, 219–229.

Warner-Smith, M., Darke, S., Lynskey, M. & Hall, W. (2001). Heroin overdose: causes and consequences. *Addiction*, *96*, 1113–1125.

Warner-Smith, M., Darke, S. & Day, C. (2002). Morbidity associated with non-fatal heroin overdose. *Addiction*, *97*, 963–967.

Weatherburn, D. & Lind, B. (2001). *Delinquent-prone Communities*. Cambridge: Cambridge University Press.

Weiss, R. D., Mirin, S. M., Griffin, M. L. & Michael, J. L. (1988). Psychopathology in cocaine abusers. Changing trends. *Journal of Nervous and Mental Disease*, *176*, 719–725.

Wells, J. E. & McGee, M. A. (2008). Violations of the usual sequence of drug initiation: prevalence and associations with the development of dependence in the New Zealand Mental Health Survey. *Journal of Studies in Alcohol and Drugs*, *69*, 789–795.

Wells, J. E., Browne, O., Scott, K. M., McGee, M. A., Baxter, J. & Kokaua, J. (2006). Prevalence, interference with life and severity of 12 month DSM-IV disorders in Te Rau Hinengaro: the New Zealand Mental Health Survey. *Australian and New Zealand Journal of Psychiatry*, *40*, 845–854.

West, R. (2005). Time for a change: putting the transtheroetical (stages of change) model to rest. *Addiction*, *100*, 1036–1039.

West, R. (2006). *Theory of Addiction*. Oxford: Addiction Press.

Westermeyer, J., Wahmanholm, K. & Thuras, P. (2001). Effects of childhood physical abuse on course and severity of substance abuse. *The American Journal on Addictions*, *10*, 101–110.

White, A. G., Birnbaum, H. G., Mareva, M. N. *et al.* (2005). Direct costs of opioid abuse in an insured population in the United States. *Journal of Managed Care Pharmacy*, *11*, 469–479.

White, A. M., Truesdale, M. C., Bae, J. G. *et al.* (2002). Differential effects of ethanol on motor coordination in adolescent and adult rats. *Pharmacology, Biochemistry and Behavior*, *73*, 673–677.

White, D. & Pitts, P. (1998). Educating young people about drugs: a systematic review. *Addiction*, *93*, 1475–1487.

White, J. & Irvine, R. (1999). Mechanisms of fatal opioid overdose. *Addiction*, *95*, 961–972.

Wilcox, H. C., Connor, K. R. & Caine, E. D. (2004). Association of alcohol and drug use disorders and completed suicide: an empirical review of cohort studies. *Drug and Alcohol Dependence, 76S*, S11–S19.

Wilens, T. E., Biedeman, J., Bredin, E. *et al.* (2002). A family study of the high-risk children of opioid- and alcohol-dependent parents. *The American Journal on Addictions, 11*, 41–51.

Wilkinson, R. & Marmot, M. (eds.) (2003). *The Solid Facts: Social Determinants of Health,* 2nd edn. Copenhagen: Centre for Urban Health, World Health Organization.

Williamson, A., Darke, S., Ross, J. & Teesson, M. (2007). Effect of baseline cocaine use on treatment outcomes for heroin dependence over 24 months. *Journal of Substance Abuse Treatment, 33*, 287–293.

Wines, J. D., Saitz, R., Horton, N. J., Lloyd-Travaglini, C. & Samet, J. (2004). Suicidal behavior, drug use and depressive symptoms after detoxification: a 2 year prospective study. *Drug and Alcohol Dependence, 76S*, S21–S29.

Wines, J. D., Saitz, R., Horton, N. J., Lloyd-Travaglini, C. & Samet, J. H. (2007). Overdose after detoxification: a prospective study. *Drug and Alcohol Dependence, 89*, 161–169.

Winick, C. (1962). Maturing out of narcotic addiction. *Bulletin on Narcotics, 14*, 1–7.

Winick, C. (1964). The life cycle of the narcotic addict and of addiction. *Bulletin on Narcotics, 16*, 1–11.

Wood, E., Tyndall, M., Zhengou, Q., Zhang, R., Montaner, J. & Kerr, T. (2006). Service uptake and characteristics of injection drug users utilizing North America's first medically supervised safer injecting facility. *American Journal of Public Health, 96*, 770–773.

Wood, E., Lloyd-Smith, E., Li, K. *et al.* (2007). Frequent needle exchange use and HIV incidence in Vancouver, Canada. *The American Journal of Medicine, 120*, 172–179.

Wu, N. S., Schairer, L. C., Dellor, E. & Grell, C. (2010). Childhood trauma and health outcomes in adults with comorbid substance abuse and mental health disorders. *Addictive Behaviors 35*, 68–71.

Yin, L., Qin, G., Ruan, Y. *et al.* (2007). Non-fatal overdose among heroin users in South-western China. *American Journal of Drug and Alcohol Abuse, 33*, 505–516.

Zaccarelli, M., Gattari, P., Rezza, G. *et al.* (1994). Impact of HIV infection on non-AIDS mortality among Italian injecting drug users. *AIDS, 8*, 345–350.

Zador, D., Lyons-Wall, P. M. & Webster, I. (1996). High sugar intake in a group of women on methadone maintenance in south western Sydney. *Addiction, 91*, 1053–1061.

Zammit, S., Allebeck, P., Andreasson, S., Lundberg, I. & Lewis, G. (2002). Self reported cannabis use as a risk factor for schizophrenia in Swedish conscripts of 1969: historical cohort study. *British Medical Journal, 325*, 1199.

Zhang, L., Ruan, Y. H., Yang, Z. N. *et al.* (2005). A 1-year prospective cohort study on mortality of injecting drug users. *Chinese Journal of Epidemiology*, 26, 190–193.

Ziedonis, D. M., Amass, L., Steinberg, M. *et al.* (2009). Predictors of outcome for short-term medically supervised opioid withdrawal during a randomized, multi center trial of buprenorphine-naloxone and clonidine in the NIDA clinical trials network. *Drug and Alcohol Dependence*, 99, 28–36.

Index

Note: page numbers in *italics* refer to tables